The Architecture of the Body and the Order of Life

Selections from Ibn Sīnā's Canon of Medicine

Ancient Wisdom Collection

Volume 2

Printed in the United States of America.

INTEGR8D.org

About the Series

The Ancient Wisdom Collection
is devoted to translating, editing, and contextualizing the foundational works of the world's great scientific and philosophical traditions.

Each volume seeks to reintroduce classical knowledge as a living intellectual system—not as relic or curiosity, but as a coherent model of inquiry that continues to inform modern thought.

Publisher's Preface

The Architecture of the Body and the Order of Life presents Ibn Sīnā's vision of the human body as an integrated system in which structure and function are inseparably joined. Beginning with the nature and classification of organs, he traces the hierarchy through which bones, tissues, and vital systems are arranged to sustain both life and motion. Each part is defined not merely by its form, but by its role—its *quwwa* (power) and *ʿamal* (action)—within a larger, ordered whole. In this account, anatomy becomes more than description; it is the study of a living architecture governed by balance (*mizāj*), coordination, and purpose, where the stability of the body and the continuity of life depend on the harmony of its parts. The selection is drawn from *Ibn Sīnā's Canon of Medicine* (*al-Qānūn fī al-Ṭibb*).

Ibn Sīnā (Avicenna, 980–1037 CE) conceived medicine as the applied art of maintaining equilibrium within the living body. To him, the physician was both a scientist and a philosopher of nature, charged not only with healing disease but with understanding the laws that govern vitality itself.

This translation presents that vision anew—faithful to his terminology, rigorous in structure, and accessible to readers of medicine, philosophy, and the sciences alike.

We invite you to immerse yourself in this selection and discover the depth and coherence of Ibn Sīnā's vision of the living body. Stay engaged as the editors of the *Ancient Wisdom Collection* continue to bring forward future volumes, each uncovering new dimensions of this enduring intellectual tradition.

Contents

Editor's Note

This second volume of *Selections from Ibn Sīnā's Canon of Medicine* continues the project begun in *The System of Nature and the Balance of Life.* Whereas the first volume explored the *architecture of the body*—its bones, joints, and muscles—this work turns to what gives that structure life: the *vital spirit* and the *networks through which it moves.*

Here, in *The Architecture of the Body and the Order of Life,* Ibn Sīnā's vision unfolds from anatomy to vitality. The reader encounters a physician-philosopher who perceived the body not as a mere assemblage of parts but as a living system animated by *energies, forces, and harmonies.* Every pulse, every breath, and every nerve current, in his account, participates in a grand *dynamic equilibrium* that sustains being and maintains life.

The text opens with the *nervous system,* through which the brain's subtle energy—the *rūḥ ḥayawānī*—flows, commanding both sensation and motion. It proceeds to the *sensory organs,* instruments of perception that bridge the material and the spiritual. From there, the discussion moves into the *vascular and nutritive systems,* where Ibn Sīnā explains how nourishment transforms into *vitality,* and how balance among the four *humors* maintains health. The volume concludes with the *reproductive and generative systems,* in which the same cosmic principles of heat, moisture, and formative power shape new life.

As with all his writings, Ibn Sīnā's synthesis in these chapters transcends his time. His concept of the body as an integrated *system of systems*—each operating through work (*ʿamal*), energy (*quwwah*), and time (*zamān*)—anticipates the frameworks of modern physiology and *systems theory.* His language of balance and temperament, though rooted in premodern cosmology, reflects a *holistic* understanding that medicine is at once physical, energetic, and moral.

This translation presents Ibn Sīnā's work in a form faithful to his style yet accessible to contemporary readers. Arabic terms of precision are transliterated, ensuring that key concepts—such as *rūḥ*, *mizāj*, *ṭabīʿa*, and *quwwa*—retain their original depth. Each section is contextualized within its intellectual lineage, linking Avicenna's insights to the continuum of Greek, Islamic, and modern thought.

The *Ancient Wisdom Collection* aims to recover not merely the texts of the past but their living systems of thought. In this spirit, *The Architecture of the Body and the Order of Life* offers a window into the enduring dialogue between body and soul, nature and order, work and equilibrium.

Editors,
Ancient Wisdom Collection

The Architecture of the Body and the Order of Life

Selections from Ibn Sīnā's Canon of Medicine

Ancient Wisdom Collection — Volume 2

The Fifth Teaching

A Single Chapter in Five Sections

On the Nature of the Organ and Its Divisions

The organs are bodies generated from the first mixture (*imtizāj*) of the well-tempered humors, just as the humors themselves are bodies generated from the first mixture of the elements. Among the organs are those that are *simple* and those that are *composite.*

A *simple organ* is that whose every sensible part, when taken separately, partakes of the same name and definition as the whole—for instance, flesh and its parts, bone and its parts, nerve and its parts, and the like. These are called *organs of homogeneous parts* (*mutashābih al-ajzā'*).

A *composite organ,* on the other hand, is one whose individual parts are not identical with the whole in name or in definition. Thus, a part of the face is not itself a face, and a portion of the hand is not a hand. Such are called *instrumental organs* (*a'ḍā' āliyya*), for they serve as the instruments of the soul in the completion of motion and action.

The first of the homogeneous organs is the *bone.* It was created firm and solid because it forms the foundation of the body and the pillar of its motions.

Next is the *cartilage* (*ghuḍrūf*), which is softer than bone so that it may bend, yet harder than most other organs. The advantage in its creation is that it mediates between the hard and the soft members: so that hard and soft are not directly joined, for in such case the soft would be harmed by the hard, especially under impact or pressure. Instead, composition proceeds by gradation—as in the shoulder bone, the sternum, and the costal cartilages at the back. The laryngeal cartilage beneath the throat is another such example.

Cartilage also facilitates the junction of moving joints, preventing their surfaces from bruising one another through their hardness. Moreover, when a muscle extends toward an organ that lacks a bony point of support—such as the muscles of the eyelids—the cartilage serves as a brace and anchor for their tendons. Likewise, in many other places the body requires some firm but not too rigid substance upon which motions depend, as in the structure of the larynx.

After cartilage comes the *nerve* (*ʿaṣab*), which arises from the brain or spinal cord. It is white, pliable, and capable of bending yet resistant to tearing. It was created to serve as the means through which the organs experience *sensation* and perform *motion.*

Next are the *tendons* (*awtār*), which grow from the ends of muscles and resemble nerves in form. They connect to the moving organs, sometimes drawing them together through the contraction of the muscle and its retraction backward, and at other times releasing them through the muscle's relaxation and extension to its natural position—or even beyond it, according to the measure of its original length. Most tendons are formed from the nerve that runs through the muscle and emerges from it on the opposite side.

Following the tendons come the *ligaments* (*rubāṭāt*), so called because they bind and join. They are also nervous in appearance and texture. They extend from various organs toward the muscles and branch into fibers along with the tendons. The portion nearest the muscle becomes filled with flesh, while the part that departs toward the joint or the movable member twists upon itself and becomes tendon-like.

Among these ligaments, some are called simply *bindings* (*ribāṭ*), while others have a special name, such as the *ʿaqb*—the thick binding at the heel. That which extends to a muscle is called a ligament, but that which connects one end of a joint's bones to another, or fastens one organ firmly to another, is also called *ʿaqb*. None of the ligaments possess sensation, for if they did, the perpetual motion and friction they endure would cause pain. Their utility, however, is evident from what has already been said: they preserve stability and coherence among the moving parts.

Then come the *arteries* (*shiryānāt*), which arise from the heart. They are elongated, hollow, nerve-like and ligamentous in substance, capable of expansion and contraction alternating with intervals of stillness. They were created to ventilate the heart, to expel its smoky vapors, and—by the permission of God—to distribute the *vital spirit* throughout the body.

The *veins* (*awrida*) resemble the arteries but originate from the liver. They are still rather than pulsating, and their purpose is to distribute *blood* to the organs of the body.

Next are the *membranes* (*aghashiya*). These are woven tissues of imperceptibly fine, nerve-like fibers, delicate in thickness and spread across the surfaces of other bodies, enveloping them for various purposes:
— To preserve the shape and integrity of each organ.
— To attach one organ to another through interlacing nerve and ligament fibers, as seen in the kidneys and spine.
— To provide for organs lacking inherent sensitivity a sensitive surface, so that they may perceive by proxy what they could not perceive by essence.

Such are the lungs, the liver, the spleen, and the kidneys. These organs in themselves are insensible; yet they perceive external impact through the membranes that envelop them. When wind or swelling occurs within them, the sensation arises indirectly: the membrane senses the stretching caused by wind, and it feels heaviness through the tension produced by swelling.

Lastly comes *flesh* (*laḥm*), which fills the spaces among these organs and serves as the medium of their strength and cohesion. Every organ possesses within itself an *innate faculty* by which nutrition is accomplished: the faculty to attract nourishment, retain it, assimilate it, attach it, and expel its residue.

Beyond this, the organs differ. Some possess, in addition to this nutritive power, another by which they act upon others; some lack that. Again, from another aspect, some possess a power by which they receive influence from another organ, while others do not. Thus, when combined, we find: an organ that both gives and receives; one that receives but does not give; one that gives but does not receive; and one that neither gives nor receives.

Of the *receptive and giving organ*, there is no doubt—both brain and liver are agreed upon as such, for each receives the power of life, innate heat, and spirit from the heart, and each in turn is a source of another power which it imparts to others.

As for the *receptive but not giving organ*, its existence is likewise clear—such as the flesh, which receives sensation and life but is not a source of power for another organ.

Concerning the *giving but not receptive organ*, the physicians and philosophers have disagreed. Many of the ancients held that this organ is the *heart*, the original source of all powers; it bestows upon the other organs all their faculties—those by which they nourish, perceive, and move. But the physicians, along with some early philosophers, distributed these powers among different organs, denying that there exists any one organ that gives without receiving. Upon close examination, the view of the ancients proves sound, though the physicians' claim appears, at first sight, more plausible.

As for the *neither-giving-nor-receiving organ*, physicians themselves differ, as do the philosophers among them. Some maintained that the bones, the insensitive flesh, and similar structures subsist through their own special powers, not derived from any other source. When nourishment reaches them, they suffice by their own nature: they impart no power to others, nor receive one in return. Others contended that these powers are not intrinsic, but were first diffused into them from the liver or the heart at the beginning of formation and have since become settled within them.

For the physician, it is not necessary to pursue by demonstration which of these views is true; the matter lies beyond his craft. His art is not harmed by either position. What he must know and acknowledge regarding the first disagreement is that, whether the heart is the source of sensation and movement for the brain and the nutritive faculty for the liver or not, it remains that the brain—either by itself or through the mediation of the heart—is the origin of the psychic actions with respect to all other organs.

On the Hierarchy of Organs and the Generation of the Body

The *liver* is likewise the origin of the *natural functions*—those that sustain nourishment and growth—in relation to all other organs. One must understand, regarding the second point of disagreement, that it makes no difference whether the *innate power* found in the bone at its first formation originates from the liver, or whether it is due to the bone's own temperament, or whether it comes from neither. What must be held now is that this power is not transmitted from the liver in such a way that, if the passage between them were blocked while nourishment still reached the bone, its action would cease—as sensation and motion cease when the nerve from the brain is obstructed. Rather, this power has become intrinsic and natural (*gharīziyya*) to the bone so long as its temperament endures.

At this point, the hierarchy of the organs becomes clear, and we may divide them into:

- *Principal organs* (*aʿḍāʾ raʾīsiyya*),
- *Servant organs* (*khādimah*),
- *Subordinate organs without service*, and
- *Organs neither principal nor subordinate.*

The *principal organs* are those that serve as the primary sources of the first powers of the body—powers necessary for the preservation either of the *individual* or of the *species.*

With respect to the preservation of the individual, there are three principal organs:

- the *heart*, the source of the vital power and life itself;
- the *brain*, the source of sensation and motion;
- and the *liver*, the source of nutrition and growth.

With respect to the preservation of the species, these three remain principal, and a fourth is added—the *testicles* (*al-unthiyān*), which are necessary for one purpose and beneficial for another. They are necessary for the *generation of semen*, through which the lineage of living beings is preserved; and they are beneficial because they perfect the male and female constitutions and temperaments—features that, though accidental, are essential to the continuation of the species, even if not to the essence of animality itself.

As for the *servant organs*, some serve through *preparatory function* (*manfaʿa*), others through *executive function* (*khidma*). The preparatory service precedes the act of the principal organ, while the executive service follows it.

Thus, the heart's preparatory servant is the *lung*, which tempers and refines the air; its executive servant is the *arterial system*, which carries the vital spirit and heat.

The brain's preparatory servant is the *liver* and other organs concerned with the maintenance and refreshment of the *spirit*; its executive servant is the *nervous system*, which conveys motion and sensation.

The liver's preparatory servant is the *stomach*, where digestion begins; its executive servant is the *venous system*, which distributes the blood it produces.

The testicles' preparatory servants are the *organs that generate semen* before it, and their executive servants in men are the *urethra* and the *vessels* between it and the testes; similarly, in women, the vessels that carry the semen to the *uterus*, where the completion of conception occurs.

Galen remarked that some organs have *function* alone, some have *benefit* alone, and others have both. The first category is exemplified by the *heart*; the second, by the *lungs*; and the third, by the *liver*.

To clarify this, we must understand by *function* (*fiʿl*) that which is performed by an organ alone, within the acts necessary for the life of the individual or the preservation of the species—such as the heart's generation of the vital spirit. By *benefit* (*manfaʿa*), we mean the condition or preparation that allows another organ's act to be perfected—such as the lung's preparation of air, without which the heart's act could not be complete.

The liver, then, performs the *second digestion* and prepares for the *third and fourth* digestions, while completing the first in such a way that the resulting blood is fit to nourish itself. Thus, it both acts (*does*) and benefits (*prepares*). At times it performs an act that is itself a benefit, in that it prepares for another act that follows it.

Furthermore, it may be said generally that among the organs, some are formed *from semen* and others *from blood*. Those of homogeneous structure—except flesh and fat—are formed from *semen*; flesh and fat are formed from *blood*. Everything else in the body originates from both the male and female semen. Yet, according to the most accurate philosophers, the embryo forms primarily from the *male semen*, in the way that *cheese* is formed from *rennet*, while the female semen plays the part of *milk*. Just as rennet initiates coagulation, so the male semen initiates the form; and just as milk provides the material that receives the coagulation, so the female semen provides the matter in which the form is established.

Each of the two, male and female semen, thus contributes part of the substance of the resulting being, as both rennet and milk are parts of the substance of cheese.

This opinion differs—indeed, diverges greatly—from that of *Galen*, who maintained that each of the two semen contains both an *active* and a *passive* power of formation. Yet it is not impossible to reconcile the views by saying that the active power is stronger in the male semen, while the receptive power is stronger in the female. The full examination of this matter, however, belongs to our works on the *natural sciences* (*al-ʿulūm al-aṣliyya*).

As for the *menstrual blood* that flows from the woman during her cycles: this becomes the *nourishment* of the embryo. Part of it is transformed into the substance resembling that of semen and the organs derived from it, thus becoming the food that sustains the embryo's growth. Another part does not serve that end but coagulates within the cavities and spaces of the primary organs, forming *flesh* and *fat*. The remainder, which is unfit for either of these uses, remains until the time of *childbirth*, when Nature expels it as surplus.

After birth, the *blood* produced by the newborn's *liver* replaces that maternal blood and performs the same functions: from it arise the same organs and tissues that had previously depended on the mother's nourishment. Flesh is generated from the *dense part* of the blood, being solidified by *heat* and *dryness.*

Fat (*shaḥm*) arises from the watery and oily portions of the blood; *cold* congeals it, which is why *heat* dissolves it. As for organs whose substance is derived from the two semens, when such an organ is severed it is rarely restored by true reunion—save in a few cases and in the years of childhood: for example, bone, and small branches of the veins, but not the large ones, nor the arteries. And if a portion of such an organ is lost, nothing grows in its stead—such is the case with *bone* and *nerve.*

By contrast, organs fashioned from *blood* regenerate after being broken or cut and join to their like—such as *flesh.* And what is generated from blood that still retains the *power of semen*: so long as the connection with semen is recent, if the part is lost it may grow again—as with a *tooth* in the years of childhood. But when another temperament gains mastery over the blood, it does not grow again.

Know also that sensitive, motive organs sometimes receive both *sensation* and *motion* from a single *nerve*; at other times the sources separate, so that each power arises from its own nerve.

All the viscera wrapped in membrane take their membranes from one of two inner linings: the lining of the *chest* and that of the *abdomen.* What lies in the chest—such as the *diaphragm,* the veins and arteries, and the *lung*—derives its membranes from the lining that coats the ribs within. What lies in the abdominal cavity—organs and vessels—derives its membranes from the *peritoneum* (*al-ṣifāq*) lining the belly's musculature.

Moreover, every fleshy organ is either *fibrous* (as the flesh of the muscles) or *without visible fibers* (as the *liver*). No movement occurs without fiber. Voluntary movements are by the fibers of *muscle.* Natural movements—such as those of the *uterus* and the *vessels*—and *compound* movements—such as *deglutition*—

proceed by a special disposition of fibers set *longitudinally*, *transversely*, and *obliquely*: longitudinal fibers for *attraction*; transverse, constricting fibers for *expulsion*; oblique fibers for *retention*.

In organs that have a *single layer*—as in the *veins*—the three kinds of fibers are woven into one another. In organs with *two layers*, the *transverse* fibers are placed in the *outer* layer, while the *longitudinal* and *oblique* are set in the *inner* layer, with the longitudinal inclined toward the inner surface. They were so created lest the fiber for *attraction* and the fiber for *expulsion* directly oppose one another; attraction and retention are better joined together—*except* in the *intestines*, whose need is not for strong retention but for attraction and expulsion.

Nervous (i.e., tendon-like) organs that surround bodies foreign to their essence are of two kinds: some have *one layer*, some *two*. Those made *double-layered* were so made for several benefits. First, where there is need of great precaution for the firmness of their substance—lest they tear under the force of the motions within, as in the *arteries*. Second, where there is need of great precaution regarding the *stored substance*, lest it *dissipate* or *escape*: dissipation would occur through thinness if the wall were single, and escape through a tendency to split. Such stored substances are the *spirit* and the *blood* contained in the arteries, whose preservation must be safeguarded: the spirit is endangered by volatilization; the blood, by rupture—both carrying grave peril.

Third, when an organ must perform both *expulsion* and *attraction* with powerful motions, each action is assigned its *own instrument* to avoid interference, as in the *stomach* and *intestines*. Fourth, when it is desired that each layer of an organ be responsible for a particular act, and the two acts arise from *contrary temperaments*, separation is sounder—*as in the stomach*: it was desired that it possess *sensation* (which belongs to a *nervous* organ) and *digestion* (which belongs to a *fleshy* organ), so a *nervous inner* layer was assigned for sensation and a *fleshy outer* layer for digestion. The inner was made nervous and the outer fleshy because the *digester* may reach the thing digested *by its power* without direct contact, whereas the *tactile sensor* cannot perceive its object except *by contact.*

There are also organs whose temperament is *near* to that of *blood.* For these, blood does not need to undergo many transformations to nourish them—such is *flesh.* Hence no cavities or recesses were made in it where arriving nourishment might abide until the flesh has fed upon it; rather, the nourishment becomes like it *as soon as it encounters it.*

Other organs are *far* in temperament from blood, and the blood must pass through *graded transformations* before it becomes like them—as with *bone.* Therefore, in their creation bone was given either a *single cavity* to hold its nourishment for the time needed for such transformation—like the bones of the *leg* and *forearm*—or *scattered cavities* within—like the bone of the *lower jaw* (*ʿaẓm al-falak al-asfal*). Organs of this sort require that nourishment be set aside *beyond the immediate need,* so that it may be converted little by little into their likeness.

Strong organs drive their *surpluses* into neighboring *weaker* parts: the *heart* to the *armpits,* the *brain* to the region *behind the ears,* and the *liver* to the *two groins* (*al-arbiyatān*).

The First Division: The Bones

(Comprising Thirty Chapters)

Chapter One: On the Bones and Joints

Among the bones, some serve in the body as *foundations* upon which its structure is built—like the *vertebrae of the spine*, which are to the body as the keel is to a ship, laid down first and supporting the whole. Some bones serve as *shields and defenses*, such as the *fontanel bone* protecting the brain. Others act as *weapons of repulsion*, driving away collision and harm—like the *spinal spines* (*sanāsin*), which project from the vertebrae like thorns. Some bones are *fillers* placed between the gaps of joints, such as the *sesamoid bones* situated between the phalanges. Others are *attachments* for organs needing points of suspension—such as the *hyoid-like bone* supporting the muscles of the larynx and the tongue.

In sum, the bones form the *support and framework* of the body. Those required solely for support or protection are *solid* (though containing necessary pores and channels). Bones also needed for *movement* are given a *central cavity*, single and unified, so that nourishment is not scattered in multiple recesses—which would make them soft—but is instead concentrated, making them dense and strong. Their nourishment lies in their *marrow*. The cavity's enlargement makes the bone *lighter*; its unity keeps it *stronger*; its firmness prevents it from breaking under violent motion; and the marrow nourishes and moistens it continually, preventing desiccation and crumbling from motion. Thus, though hollow, the bone remains like a solid body.

Where strength is more necessary, the cavity is smaller; where lightness is needed, it is greater. The *spongy bones* (*ʿiẓām mushāshiyya*) were formed thus not only for nourishment but also for special purposes—such as allowing passage for inhaled *odors* through the *ethmoid bone,* and to receive the *surplus vapors* expelled from the brain.

All bones are adjacent and contiguous. Between one bone and another there is little distance, and what space exists is filled with *cartilaginous* or *cartilage-like* tissues that serve the functions of cartilage. Where no such utility is required, the *joint* (*mafṣil*) is formed directly between the bones, as in the *lower jaw.*

The contiguity between bones takes several forms. Some joints are *loose and free-moving*; some *stiff but unfastened*; others *firmly fixed*—either *inserted, sutured,* or *adhered.*

The *free joint* is that in which one bone can move easily without moving the other—like the joint of the *wrist* with the *forearm.* The *stiff, unfastened joint* is one in which the movement of one bone alone is difficult and of small range, as between the *carpus and metacarpus* or between two *metacarpal bones.* The *fixed joint* is that in which neither bone moves independently—like the *sternal joints.*

The *inserted joint* is that in which one bone has a *projection* and the other a *socket* in which that projection is set firmly, immovably—like the *teeth* in their sockets.

The *sutured joint* is where both bones have *notches and ridges,* interlocked like the teeth of a saw, each ridge fitting into the notch of the other, as *smiths* join sheets of metal. This joint is called *suture* (*darz*), as in the *cranial sutures.*

The *adhering joint* may be *longitudinal*—as between the *bones of the forearm*—or *transverse,* as between the *lower vertebrae* of the spine, for the upper vertebrae are not tightly fixed.

Chapter Two: The Anatomy of the Skull (al-Qaḥf)

The skull's general purpose is to *protect and shelter the brain* from harm. Its structure, composed of many bones and sections, serves two sets of functions:

(1) those pertaining to the *bone itself*, and
(2) (2) those pertaining to what the bone *contains.*

Regarding the first: the multiplicity of cranial bones ensures that when one part suffers fracture or decay, the defect is not transmitted to the whole, as would happen if it were a single solid bone. It also allows variation in thickness, density, and strength within the same structure, corresponding to functional needs.

As for the second: the skull's apertures and sutures serve several purposes. Some relate to the *brain itself*—providing passages through which *vapors* may escape when they cannot penetrate the bone's dense substance, thereby *purifying* the brain. Others serve as outlets for the *nerves* that arise from the brain to supply the head's organs. Two functions are shared between the brain and other structures: one for the *veins and arteries* entering the cranial cavity, giving them passage; another for the *thick dura mater*, parts of which attach to the sutures, preventing it from weighing upon the brain.

The skull's natural shape is *rounded*, serving two purposes. Internally, the sphere encloses the largest possible space for a given surface area; externally, it best resists impact, being less affected by blows than angular forms. It is somewhat *elongated*, because the origins of the cranial nerves are arranged lengthwise; and this elongation also prevents compression. It bears *projections* at the front and back to shield the nerves descending from either side.

There are *three true sutures* and *two false.*

The first true suture is the *coronal* (*iklīlī*), arching across the head like a diadem and joining the frontal bone.

The second is the *sagittal* (*sahmī*), running lengthwise through the middle of the skull, sometimes called *safūdī* when considered in relation to the coronal, its shape resembling a bow with a straight line through its center.

The third is the *lambdoid suture* (*lāmī*), shared between the back of the skull and its base, shaped like an angle whose vertex meets the end of the sagittal suture, named for its resemblance to the Greek letter *lambda (Λ).*

The two *false sutures* run lengthwise along both sides, parallel to the sagittal, shallowly grooved and therefore called *cortical sutures* (*qashariyyān*).

Abnormal skull shapes are three:

(1) where the *anterior projection* is deficient, losing part of the coronal suture;

(2) where the *posterior projection* is deficient, losing part of the lambdoid; and

(3) where *both* projections are absent, yielding a *globular head* equal in length and breadth.

Galen, the most eminent of physicians, held that when the skull's dimensions are equal, the sutures must likewise be proportioned: originally there were three—one longitudinal and two transverse—but in the globular form there are but two, one for each dimension, with the transverse stretching from *ear to ear* and the longitudinal from *front to back.*

He further asserted that no *fourth natural shape* of the skull exists. A head shorter than its breadth would diminish the volume or substance of the brain, a condition incompatible with life and sound composition. Thus, he affirmed the correctness of *Hippocrates*, who had reduced the natural shapes of the head to four.

Chapter Three: Anatomy of What Lies Beneath the Skull

Below the cranial vault are *five bones*: four forming the *walls* and one forming the *base*. The walls are made *denser* than the *fontanel* bones, for they are more exposed to *falls and blows*; the fontanel, by contrast, requires *porosity* for two reasons—so that vapors from within may escape, and so that it may not weigh heavily upon the brain.

- The *posterior wall* is the *strongest*, since it is least guarded by the senses.
- The *first wall* is the *frontal bone*, bounded above by the *coronal suture* and below by another extending from one end of the coronal, passing above the eye along the *brow*, and joining the opposite end of the same.

The *two lateral walls*—those containing the *ears*—are the *temporal bones*, called the *chambers* (*ḥujratān*) for their hardness. Each is bounded above by the *cortical suture*, below by a line running from the *lambdoid* to the *coronal*, and anteriorly and posteriorly by portions of those same sutures.

The *fourth wall* is bounded above by the *lambdoid suture* and below by the *joint between the skull and the wedge-shaped bone (al-watadī)*, connecting the two ends of the lambdoid.

The *base of the brain* rests upon the *sphenoid bone* (*al-ʿaẓm al-watadī*), which supports all the cranial bones. It was made hard for two reasons: first, because hardness aids in bearing weight; second, because what is dense resists corruption better. This bone lies directly beneath the region where impurities and waste descend continually; hence, its firmness serves as protection.

On each side of the *temples* are two other solid bones that cover the *nerve* passing through the temple. They are set obliquely along its length and are called *the pair (az-zawj).*

Chapter Four: Anatomy of the Bones of the Jaws and the Nose

As for the bones of the jaw and the temple, their number is clarified by tracing the sutures of the jaw. The *upper jaw* is bounded above by a suture shared with the frontal bone, running beneath the brow from temple to temple; below, by the line of the tooth-sockets; and on both sides by a buttressing suture coming from the region of the ear, shared with the *wedge-shaped* bone (*al-ʿaẓm al-watadī,* the sphenoid) that lies behind the molars. Its far end inclines slightly inward, so that a suture divides it from another suture that runs lengthwise across the roof of the palate. These are its outer limits.

Within these limits there are internal sutures: one that cuts the roof of the palate lengthwise; a second that begins between the eyebrows and descends to the midline between the two central incisors; a third that starts where the second begins, then slopes down to the line between the right lateral incisor and the canine; and a fourth, symmetrical on the left. Thus there are three central sutures with two lateral limits. Between these three central sutures and the line of the tooth-sockets lie two *triangular bones.* The bases of these triangles do not sit exactly at the tooth-sockets, for a transverse suture intervenes near the base of the nostrils. The three central sutures pass beyond this transverse line to the places described. Below the two triangles lie two other bones encompassed together by the bases of the triangles, the tooth-sockets, and parts of the lateral sutures. A descending branch from the middle suture separates these two bones, so that each has two right angles along this dividing line, an acute angle at the canine, and an obtuse angle near the nostril.

Among the sutures of the upper jaw is another descending from the superior common suture toward the orbit. When it reaches the *orbital fossa*, it divides into three branches: one passes beneath the suture shared with the frontal bone and above the fossa until it meets the brow; a second, slightly lower, reaches the same destination without entering the fossa; and a third reaches it after entering the fossa. The lower the branch relative to the brow suture, the farther it runs from its point of contact with the upper. The bone set off by the *first* of these three is the largest, then that separated by the second.

The *nose* has three manifest benefits. First, by means of its cavity, it assists *inspiration*: air gathers within it in greater quantity and is moderated before passing inward, for although inhaled air goes to the lungs, a sizeable portion also reaches the brain. The nose likewise concentrates, for purposes of *olfaction*, an appropriate volume of air in front of the organ of smell, making perception stronger and more precise—three utilities encompassed in one. Second, it aids the *articulation of speech*, easing the emission of letters so that the breath does not crowd all at once at the points of articulation; here its function resembles that of the opening behind the glottis, which must not be obstructed. Third, it serves as a *cover and screen* for the discharges descending from the head and as an instrument to *expel* them by blowing.

The nasal bones are two triangles whose upper angles meet; their bases touch at one corner and separate at the other two. Each rests on one of the two lateral sutures described beneath the facial suture. On their inferior outer edges lie two soft cartilages, and between them, along the median suture, a *middle cartilage* whose upper part is firmer than its lower and which is, overall, firmer than the two lateral cartilages. The middle cartilage divides the nose into two *nostrils* so that descending humors from the brain, when they fall, incline mostly to one side, and do not block the entire passage by which ventilating air—bearing *spirit*—ascends to the brain. The two lateral cartilages have three purposes: they share the general benefit of cartilages placed at bony extremities (already mentioned); they allow the alae to *dilate* when greater inspiration or forceful blowing is needed; and, by their vibration in blowing, they *break up vapors* and help expel them.

The nasal bones were made *thin and light* because lightness is more needed here than solidity, especially since they are not tasked with bearing or transmitting forces from organs liable to injury and are placed under the constant surveillance of the senses.

The *lower jaw* has fewer bones and an evident function. It consists of two bones joined beneath the chin by a *firm joint*; each bone then spreads backward, ending in an elevated, hooked process that articulates with a shaped eminence at the cranial base, the two held together by strong *ligaments*.

Chapter Five: Anatomy of the Teeth

The teeth are *thirty-two* in number, though in some persons the *third molars* (*nawājidh*, "wisdom teeth")—the four most posterior—are absent, yielding *twenty-eight*. There are *two central incisors* and *two lateral incisors* above and the like below, for cutting; *two canines* above and two below, for tearing; and *molars* for grinding—*four or five* on each side above and below. The total is therefore thirty-two or, without the wisdom teeth, twenty-eight. The wisdom teeth usually erupt toward the *middle of the growth period*, which is after the attainment of full stature, for completion is near thirty years; hence they are called the *teeth of maturity*.

Teeth have *roots* and *sharpened crowns* seated in the *alveoli* of the jawbones. Around the rim of each alveolus is a circular *bony lip* encasing and strengthening the tooth, with strong *periodontal ligaments*. Every tooth other than the molars has a *single crown.* The *lower molars* have at least *two cusps*, and the wisdom teeth often *three*; the *upper molars* have at least *three cusps*, and the wisdom teeth often *four*. The molars have many cusps because of their size and the greater work they perform; the upper have more than the lower because they are *suspended*, and the forces of mastication incline opposite the direction of their cusps, whereas the weight of the lower does not counter their seating.

No bone in the body possesses *sensation—except the teeth.* Galen says: experience itself bears witness that they feel, aided by a power supplied from the brain, so that they discern *heat and cold.*

Chapter Six: The Spine (al-Ṣulb)

The *spine* was created for *four purposes.*

First, it serves as a *channel for the spinal cord (al-nukhāʿ),* which is indispensable for the animal's life—as will be explained in detail later when discussing the marrow. Here it suffices to state generally that if *all the nerves* originated directly from the *brain*, the head would have to be far larger than it is, making it heavy and burdensome to the body. Moreover, the nerves would have to travel great distances to reach the extremities, exposing them to injury and breakage; their excessive length would also weaken their power to draw and move the heavier limbs. Thus the Creator, exalted be His name, in His wisdom caused a *portion of the brain* to extend downward like a *stream from a spring*—this is the *spinal cord*—to distribute the nerves throughout the body, according to their alignment and proximity to the organs. The spine was therefore made as a *secure conduit* to protect this vital substance.

Second, the spine serves as a *shield and protection* for the noble organs situated before it; hence, it was formed with *spines and projections* (the spinous processes).

Third, the spine forms the *main support* upon which the body's entire skeletal system is built, as the first timber set in a ship's keel, upon which the rest of the planks are fixed; thus, the spine was made firm and hard.

Fourth, the spine gives the *human form stability and erect posture*, allowing independent bearing and flexible movement in all directions. For this reason, it was not made as one solid bone, nor as many small bones, but as a *series of articulated vertebrae.* The joints between them are neither too loose—lest the body's frame become weak—nor too rigid—lest bending be prevented.

Chapter Seven: The Anatomy of the Vertebrae

A *vertebra* is a bone containing in its center a *foramen* through which the *spinal cord* passes. Each vertebra may have *four processes*—two on each side of the foramen—those projecting upward are called *superior processes*, those pointing downward are *inferior* or *inverted* ones. Sometimes there are *six processes* (four lateral and two central), and occasionally *eight.*

The purpose of these *processes* is to establish *articulated connections* among the vertebrae, each joining by *depressions* and *condyloid heads.* Other processes exist not for articulation but for *protection, defense,* and *resistance* against external blows, as well as for the attachment of *ligaments.* These are broad, solid extensions running along the spine's length. The ones placed posteriorly are called *spines* (*shuʿūk, sanāsin*), and those lateral to the axis are called *wings* (*ajniḥa*).

Their purpose is to guard the deeper structures along the body's axis—the *nerves, vessels,* and *muscles.* Some of the lateral processes, especially those that correspond to the ribs, have a special function: they bear *pits* or *depressions* for the *articulation of the rib heads,* which fit into them in a convex manner. Each *wing* (transverse process) bears *two small pits,* and each *rib* has *two convex projections.* Some wings are *double-headed,* resembling *bifid processes*, as in the *cervical vertebrae*—a structure whose benefit will be mentioned later.

Besides the main foramen for the spinal cord, the vertebrae also have *other openings* through which *nerves emerge* and *vessels enter*. Some of these apertures lie entirely within a single vertebra; others are shared between two, located at their *junction*. This may occur above, below, or on one side; in some cases, each vertebra contributes a *half-circle*, in others, one provides a larger portion than the other.

These foramina were placed *laterally* rather than *posteriorly*, because openings at the back would not be well protected and would be vulnerable to impact; nor were they placed *anteriorly*, for that region bears the *natural weight of the body* and the *strain of movement*, which would weaken the vertebrae and compress the emerging nerves.

The *protective processes* are surrounded by *ligaments and connective tissues* covered with *moist membranes*, ensuring smoothness and reducing friction, so they do not injure adjacent muscles. The *articulating processes* are also bound tightly by interlacing ligaments on all sides—though the front connections are *stronger* and the posterior ones *looser*, because forward bending is needed more frequently than backward extension.

Where the ligaments are more relaxed behind, a small *space* remains, filled with *viscous moisture* to lubricate motion. Thus, the vertebral column, by the tightness of its anterior bindings, behaves like a *single solid bone*—stable and firm; yet, by the looseness of its posterior joints, it remains as *multiple bones*—flexible and capable of motion.

Chapter Eight: The Function of the Neck and the Anatomy of Its Bones

The *neck* was created to serve the *trachea (qaṣabat al-ri'ah),* and the trachea itself was fashioned for the purposes that will be explained in its proper place.

Because the *cervical vertebrae*—indeed, the upper vertebrae in general—are supported by what lies beneath them in the *spinal column*, they were necessarily made *smaller and lighter*. For in the natural order, that which is carried must be lighter than that which carries it, if movement is to remain balanced and well-ordered.

Since the *upper portion of the spinal cord* is the *largest and thickest,* like the source of a river—because the number of nerves branching from its higher part is greater than those that emerge below—it was necessary that the *foramina* (openings) in the cervical vertebrae be *broader*. And because this broadness, coupled with the vertebrae's small size, would make their substance thin, there was need for a compensating *firmness and solidity.* Thus the cervical vertebrae were created of *dense and resilient bone.*

Their *spinous processes* were made *short,* for if they were large, the vertebrae—being delicate—would be prone to fracture upon collision with hard objects. To balance this, their *transverse processes* (wings) were made *large and bifid* (double-headed).

Because the neck needs *mobility* more than *rigidity*—for its small number of bones does not compromise stability as much as in the lower spine—the *joints* between its vertebrae were made *looser* than those below. Whatever firmness is lost by this looseness is compensated by the many *muscles, nerves, and vessels* surrounding and binding the region.

Hence, the *articular processes* of the cervical vertebrae were made *longer and narrower*, with *softer ligaments*, rather than broad and massive as in the lower vertebrae. The *nerve exits* are shared between each two vertebrae, since the small size and large central canal of each vertebra leave no space for independent openings—except in certain cases that will be described.

There are *seven cervical vertebrae*, a number perfectly suited for balance in length and function. Each, except the first, possesses *eleven processes*: one *spinous process*, two *wings*, eight *articular processes* (four upward, four downward), and each wing divided into *two branches*. The *nerve opening* between each pair of vertebrae is *shared equally*.

The *first* and *second* cervical vertebrae, however, have *unique properties*.

The First Cervical Vertebra (al-Kharza al-Ūlā)

The movement of the *head to the right and left* occurs by means of the *joint between the skull and the first vertebra*; movement *forward and backward* occurs by the *joint between the first and the second*.

The first vertebra has *two superior depressions* into which *two projections* from the skull fit. When one projection rises and the other sinks, the head inclines toward the sunken side. The second joint could not be placed upon this same vertebra, so a separate bone—the *second cervical vertebra*—was created for it.

From the *anterior part* of the second vertebra arises a *long, strong projection* that passes through an *opening in the first vertebra*, in front of the spinal cord. This shared opening is longer *front-to-back* than *side-to-side*, because it must accommodate both the passage of the *spinal canal* and the *process (tooth)* of the second vertebra.

This *process* is called the *tooth (al-sinn)*. Strong *ligaments* were formed between it and the spinal cord, separating the two so that the motion of the tooth would not crush or press upon the cord. The tooth of the second vertebra rises through the foramen of the first and fits into a *socket of the skull*, allowing the *forward and backward motion* of the head.

This projection faces *forward* for two reasons: first, for *greater protection*; and second, to ensure that the *thinner side* of the vertebra lies inward, not outward.

The first vertebra lacks a *spinous process*—so as not to burden or endanger it, for any projecting structure that defends against force can also transmit force to weaker parts and cause injury. The neck's *muscles and nerves* are thickly gathered around it, leaving little need for a bony spur; moreover, it lies *deeply protected* by surrounding tissues. For the same reason, it also lacks *transverse wings*, since there is no space for them near the origin of so many structures.

The *nerves* emerging from this vertebra exit *not from its sides* nor from a *shared opening*, but from *two small posterior apertures*—one on each side—because if they emerged near the articulations with the skull, the motion of the head would injure them.

The Second Cervical Vertebra (al-Kharza al-Thāniya)

The *tooth-like process* (odontoid) of the second vertebra is joined firmly to the first by *ligaments*, while the *joint of the skull with the first vertebra* and that of the *first and second together* are the *most flexible* in the spine, due to the necessity of extensive head movement.

When the head moves *forward or backward*, the first vertebra moves with the skull as though they were one bone. When it moves *side to side*, both the first and second vertebrae move together as one unit.

Chapter Nine: The Vertebrae of the Chest (Thoracic Vertebrae)

The *thoracic vertebrae* are those to which the *ribs* are attached, enclosing the organs of *respiration*. They number *twelve*: *eleven* with *spinous and transverse processes*, and *one (the twelfth)* without wings.

Their *spinous processes* are unequal in size: those adjacent to the *more noble organs* (such as the heart) are *larger and stronger*. Their *transverse processes* are *thicker and denser* than those elsewhere, to secure the attachment of the ribs. The *upper seven* thoracic vertebrae have *large spinous processes* and *broad wings* for thorough protection of the heart. Because of this bulk, their *articular processes* were made *short and wide*.

Above the *tenth vertebra*, the *upper articular processes* contain *pits (nukr)* for receiving the heads of adjoining bones, while the *lower ones* bear *rounded protrusions (laqam)* that fit into these pits. The *tenth vertebra's* spinous process is erect and domed, with its articular surfaces on both sides bearing *pits without protrusions*—for it articulates both above and below.

Below the *tenth*, the arrangement reverses: the *upper surfaces* have protrusions, and the *lower* have pits, and their spinous processes curve *upward*.

The *twelfth vertebra* lacks *transverse wings* because the ribs end there and their protective function is no longer needed. Yet nature compensated for this by shaping its structure to serve both *support and protection*: its *articular processes* were *doubled* and broadened, achieving the stability otherwise provided by the missing wings. This vertebra also connects with the *diaphragm*.

The thoracic vertebrae are *larger* than the cervical, so their *nerve foramina* are not perfectly divided between adjacent vertebrae. Instead, they shift gradually—slightly higher above, slightly lower below—until the *tenth vertebra*, where the openings are contained entirely within one bone. In the *lumbar vertebrae*, the openings lie wholly within each vertebra and are paired—one on the right and one on the left—for the exit of the *nerves*.

Chapter Ten: The Lumbar Vertebrae (al-Qaṭn)

The *lumbar vertebrae* bear *spinous processes* and *broad transverse processes (wings)*. Their *inferior articular processes* are flared laterally so that they resemble protective wings. They are *five* in number. Together with the *sacrum*, the loins form the *base of the entire spine*: they are its *buttress*, the *support of the pubic bone*, and the *origin of the nerves of the lower limb*.

Chapter Eleven: The Sacrum (al-ʿAjz)

The *sacrum* consists of *three* vertebrae. They are the most *firmly interlocked* of all, with the *strongest joints* and the *broadest wings*. The *nerves* leave it through *openings that are not strictly on the lateral sides*, so that they are not crowded by the *hip joint*; rather, the outlets lie *inward* and are directed *anteriorly and posteriorly*. In their general character these sacral bones resemble those of the *loins*.

Chapter Twelve: The Coccyx (al-ʿUṣʿuṣ)

The *coccyx* is composed of *three cartilaginous* segments without processes. Nerves arise from it through *shared openings*—as in the *neck*—owing to its small size; from the *third* segment a *single nerve* emerges from its tip.

Chapter Thirteen: General Conclusion on the Function of the Spine

We have spoken moderately concerning the bones of the spine; let us now give a *comprehensive statement* about the *whole.*

As a whole, the *spinal column* is fashioned with the *best of forms*, the *rounded (arched) profile*, for this is the shape least susceptible to injury from impacts. Thus the *upper spinous processes* curve *downward*, the *lower* curve *upward*, and they *meet around the middle*, at the *tenth vertebra*. That vertebra is the *middle* of the spinous processes not in *number* but in *length.*

Because the spine must *bend and incline to the sides*, its middle must be able to *shift slightly to the opposite direction*, while the parts above and below *incline toward the side of movement.* Since the two ends tend by nature to *approach one another* in such movements, the *tenth vertebra* was not provided with *convex bosses (loqam)* but with *sockets (nuqar)*; the *upper bosses* above and the *lower bosses* below were *oriented toward it.* The *upper edges* that face it are *sloped downward*, and the *lower edges* that face it are *sloped upward*—so that the middle can more easily *yield opposite the direction of the bend*: the upper part can be drawn *downward* and the lower part can be drawn *upward.*

Chapter Fourteen: The Ribs (al-Aḍlāʿ) and the Sternum (al-Qaṣ)

The *ribs* are the *armor* of the organs they enclose—*the instruments of respiration* and the *upper organs of nutrition.* They were not made a *single bone*, lest they be too heavy, lest a *single injury* ruin all, and so that the *chest* could *expand* beyond its natural resting breadth when the need for air increases or when the *viscera* are distended by food and wind. Their separateness also allows the *intercostal muscles* to interleave and assist the *acts of breathing* and related motions.

Because the chest surrounds the *lungs, heart,* and their associates, it required *the greatest care* in protection. Yet complete fortification had to avoid *constriction*. Therefore the *upper seven ribs* on each side *encircle fully* what they guard and *meet the sternum,* enclosing the principal organ on all sides.

By contrast, the ribs adjacent to the *organs of nutrition* (liver, spleen, etc.) were made like *prongs* posteriorly—where the eye does not watch—and do *not meet anteriorly*. Instead they *gradually shorten* toward the bottom, so that the *upper of these lower ribs* lies *nearest* to the sternum and the *lowest* lies *farthest*. This both protects the organs of nutrition and *widens the space of the stomach,* so it is not compressed when distended by food or wind.

Thus the *upper seven* on each side are called the *thoracic (true) ribs*. The *middle pair* among them are the *largest and longest,* and the *end pairs* are *shorter*; this configuration best *encloses* what it surrounds. Each rib first *descends with its convexity downward,* then *returns upward* to meet the sternum—so that the enclosure has the *widest capacity*.

Each rib carries *two tubercles* that fit into *two deep sockets* on each *transverse process* of the vertebrae, forming a *double articulation*; likewise the *upper seven* articulate doubly *with the sternum*.

The *remaining five*—the *shorter* ribs—belong to the *posterior chest* and are called the *false (floating/costal) ribs*. Their *anterior heads* are joined to *cartilage,* to avoid fracture in blows and so that they do not strike soft organs and the *diaphragm* with hardness, but rather with a *medium substance*—intermediate between bone and soft tissue.

The Sternum (al-Qaṣ). The *sternum* consists of *seven bones.* It is not one piece, for the same reasons stated elsewhere: to lighten weight and to assist the surrounding *respiratory organs* in their *subtle expansions*. Hence it is *slightly spongy* and joined by *cartilages* that aid its *minute motions*, even though its joints are *securely bound*. They are *seven* to match the *seven true ribs* that attach to it. At its *lower end* is a *broad cartilaginous bone* with a *rounded tip*, called the *xiphoid (al-khanjari, "dagger-shaped")* because it resembles a dagger. It *guards the mouth of the stomach* and serves as a *buffer* between sternum and soft organs, improving the *transition from hard to soft*—as we have often said.

Chapter Fifteen: The Clavicle (al-Tarqūwah)

On each side, a *clavicle* is set upon the *upper sternum*. By its *anterior convexity* it leaves at the *suprasternal notch* a *passage* for the *vessels ascending to the brain* and the *nerves descending from it*. It then *curves outward* to meet the *acromial end of the scapula*, thereby *linking the shoulder*; together with the shoulder it *suspends the arm*.

Chapter Sixteen: The Scapula (al-Katf)

The *scapula* serves *two purposes*:

1. To *hang the arm* from it, so that the *humerus* is not fixed to the chest—thus preserving the *freedom and breadth of motion* of each hand without the other becoming cramped.

2. To provide a *stout shield* for the organs within the chest, taking the place of *spinous and transverse processes* in a region where there are no vertebrae to resist blows and where no immediate sense organs would perceive them.

The scapula *tapers* toward its *lateral* end and *thickens* inward, producing at its lateral angle a *shallow socket* into which the *rounded head of the humerus* fits.

It has *two projections*:

- One *above and posteriorly*—the *acromion* (and *coracoid, "raven's beak"*)—by which the *scapula is bound to the clavicle*, preventing the *humerus* from dislocating *upward.*
- Another *medially and inferiorly*, also hindering the *head of the humerus* from dislocating.

Medially the bone *broadens*, increasing its protective *coverage*. On its dorsal surface is a *triangular spine*, with its *base lateral* and its *apex medial*, so that the *back remains flat*: were the base medial, the skin would *tent* and be *painful* in impacts. This spine is the scapula's analogue to a *spinous process*, made for *protection*, and is called the *spine of the scapula*. The lateral end of the scapula finishes in an *articular cartilage* with a *rounded margin*.

Chapter Seventeen: The Humerus (ʿAẓm al-ʿAḍud)

The *humerus* is *cylindrical*, the shape least vulnerable to impacts. Its *upper end* is *convex* and fits the *glenoid cavity* of the scapula in a *loose joint*. Because of this looseness, *dislocation* occurs frequently; yet this looseness serves *two ends*:

- **Need:** *Freedom of movement* in *all directions*.
- **Safety:** Though many motions are possible, they *do not crowd upon the humerus continually* so as to *overstretch its ligaments*, for in most tasks the *humerus rests* while the *forearm and hand* are active. Hence the other joints of the limb were *bound more firmly* than the shoulder.

The shoulder joint is secured by *four ligaments*:

1. A *capsular membrane* encircling the joint (as in other joints);

2. Two bands descending from the *acromion*: one *transverse* embracing the *head* of the humerus; the second *larger and stronger*, descending together with

3. A *fourth* band from the *nearby coracoid*, both passing in a *prepared groove* and *broadening* especially where they contact the humerus. These deeper bands *underrun the humerus* and *blend with the muscles* layered upon its inner surface.

The shaft of the humerus is *concave medially* and *convex laterally*, to receive and guide the *stacked muscles, nerves, and vessels*, to ease *carrying under the arm*, and to allow *one hand to turn toward the other.*

At the *distal end* are *two contiguous projections*. The one *medial/internal* is *longer and thinner* and *forms no joint*—it serves to *protect nerves and vessels*. The *lateral/external* one completes the *elbow joint* with a *trochlear/capitellar surface* as described below. Between the two lies a *groove*, with *two fossae*: *an anterior medial fossa*, smooth and even, and a *larger lateral fossa* whose *medial edge* is *not smooth or rounded*, but like a *straight wall*, so that when the *ulnar projection* swings outward and reaches it, it *stops*. (Hippocrates calls these two fossae the *"two eyes."*)

Chapter Eighteen: The Forearm (al-Sāʿid)

The *forearm* consists of *two bones* closely apposed along their length, called the *two zinds (ulnae/radii)*. The *upper (thumb-side)* is *slender* and called the *upper zind*; the *lower (little-finger side)* is *thicker* because it *bears weight*, and is called the *lower zind*.

- The *upper bone* provides the motions of *pronation and supination* (twisting over and back).

- The *lower bone* provides the motions of *flexion and extension*.

Each bone has a *slender middle*—since the surrounding *thick muscles* supply the needed mass without burdening the limb—and *thickened ends* to receive *strong ligamental bindings*, for these ends endure *frequent strains and impacts*, and the bones there are comparatively *bare of muscle.*

The *upper (radial) bone* is *slightly curved*, beginning medially, then *gently turning laterally in a spiral*—a shape well-suited to *twisting motion*. The *lower (ulnar) bone* is *straight*, a form best suited to *flexion and extension.*

Chapter Twenty: The Elbow Joint (al-Mirfaq)

The *elbow* is formed by the union of the *upper zind* and *lower zind* with the *humerus.*

- At its proximal end, the **upper zind** bears a *shaped socket* that receives the *lateral condyle* of the humerus; *rotation within this socket* produces *pronation and supination.*
- The **lower zind** has *two flanges* separated by a *groove shaped like the Greek sigma (ς)*. The *humeral end* that meets this groove is *concave like a rounded boss*. By the *interlocking* of the lower zind's groove with the humeral surface, the **hinge of the elbow** is completed.

When the *groove* moves *backward and downward*, the *forearm extends*; when the *groove* is checked by the *bony wall* of the receiving fossa, *further extension is prevented* and humerus and forearm come into *straight alignment*. When one *flange* slides *forward and upward* upon the other, the forearm *flexes* until the *medial and anterior* sides of forearm and arm *meet*.

Distally, the *two zinds* converge like *a unified piece* and present a *broad shared fossa*, mostly on the *lower zind*; the remainder stays *convex and polished* to ward off injury. Behind this fossa on the lower zind rises a *long posterior process*—its function will be explained presently.

Chapter Twenty-One: The Wrist (al-Rusrugh)

The *wrist* is composed of *many bones* so that *one mishap* will not ruin the whole. There are seven principal carpal bones plus one additional bone.

- The proximal row (nearest the forearm) has three bones, being the *finer* row befitting its nearness to the forearm.
- The distal row (toward the palm) has four bones, *broader* to suit their continuity with the *metacarpus and digits.*

Across the proximal row, the ends *nearest the forearm* are *slimmer* and *more tightly interlocked*; the ends *toward the distal row* are *broader* and *less interlocked.* The eighth bone does not belong to either row; it was formed to *protect a nerve* that runs along the *ulnar side of the hand.*

The *three proximal carpal bones*, by the meeting of their distal heads, form a *single convex surface* that fits into the *shared fossa* at the distal ends of the two zinds—thereby creating the joint for *flexion and extension.* The *long posterior process* on the *lower zind* fits a *socket* in the adjacent carpal bone, providing the joint for *pronation and supination.*

Chapter Twenty-Two: The Metacarpus (Mashṭ al-Kaff)

The *metacarpus* likewise is *multi-ossous*, so a single lesion does not disable the hand; its arrangement also allows the *palm to hollow* when grasping *spheres* and to *control fluids.* These bones are firmly bound, so that even if the palm's skin were removed, the *metacarpals would remain joined*, their separations remote from sensation; yet the ligatures allow a *slight yielding*—enough to *cup the palm.*

There are four metacarpal bones, one for each of the four fingers. They are *close-set* at the *carpal* end (to meet compact wrist bones) and *slightly splayed* toward the *digits* (to meet diverging phalanges). Their *palmar surfaces* are *concave* for the reasons given. The *carpo-metacarpal* joints are formed by *sockets* in the distal carpal row receiving *cartilage-clad heads* of the metacarpals.

Chapter Twenty-Three: The Digits (al-Aṣābiʿ)

The *fingers* are instruments of *grasp*. They were not made of mere flesh—lest their actions be *feeble*—nor of a *single bone*, which would make movements *awkward*. They consist of three phalanges each:

- Adding *more* would multiply directions of motion but *weaken* the grip;
- Making *fewer* would *over-stiffen* them and diminish the *range* required for dexterous tasks.

Their *bases* are *broad*, their *tips fine*; the *proximal phalanges* are *larger* by degrees, down to the *slender fingertips*. Thus the *bearer* (proximal) is proportioned to the *borne* (distal). The phalanges are *round in section* to resist blows; *solid* without *marrow cavities* for *steadfastness* in gripping and drawing. Each is *concave on the palmar side* and *convex dorsally* to improve *purchase* and *kneading/pressing*.

No general concavity/convexity was placed *between adjacent fingers*, so that together they may act as *one broad surface* when needed; yet the *outer edges* of *thumb* and *little finger* were given *lateral curvature*, so that when the hand closes the digits and palm *approximate a circle*, a shape that *defends from impacts*.

Within, the digits are *fleshy* on the palmar aspect to *buttress* and *yield* under contact; not so dorsally, lest they become *heavy* and always *injurious*. The *pulp of the fingertips* is *plentiful*, so that the ends *bed neatly* against one another in full flexion.

The *middle finger* has the *longest* phalanges, then the *ring finger*, then the *index*, then the *little finger*, so that their *tips align* in grasp without gaps while the *four fingers* and the *palm* curve together around a *round object*. The *thumb* stands as the *counter-seal* to all the rest; placed otherwise it would lose its use—set *in the palm* it would deprive us of palmar acts; set by the *little finger*, the two hands could not *face one another* well in joint grasp; set *posteriorly*, its use would be more remote still. The thumb is *not fused* to the metacarpus, lest the *distance* between it and the other digits be cramped; when the four enclose an object on one side and the thumb *opposes* from the other, the hand can *embrace a large thing*. The thumb acts as a *stopper* upon what the hand encloses; the *little* and *ring* fingers act like a *lower cover*.

All interphalangeal joints are *tongue-and-groove* (boss-and-socket) articulations, lined with *viscid moisture*, wrapped by *strong ligaments*, faced by *cartilaginous pads*; tiny *sesamoid bones* fill the *gaps* to add *security*.

Chapter Twenty-Four: The Nail (al-Ẓufr)

The *nail* serves *four purposes*:

1. *Backing* the fingertip so it does not *weaken* when pressing;
2. Enabling the finger to *pick up very small things*;
3. *Cleaning and scratching*;
4. Serving as a *weapon* at times (more for *other animals* than for humans).

Its tip is *rounded*; its substance is a *pliant bone* that *yields* under impact and does not *splinter*. Nails are *continually renewed*, for they are subject to *friction and wear*.

Chapter Twenty-Five: The Pelvic Bones (ʿiẓām al-ʿānah)

Beside the *sacrum* lie two great bones, *right and left*, meeting in the *midline* by a *firm joint*. They are as a *foundation* for all the *upper bones* and the *carriers and conveyors* of those below. Each divides into four parts:

- *Lateral/superior*: the ilium (*ḥurqafah*, "flank bone");
- *Anterior*: the pubis (*ʿaṇah*);
- *Posterior*: the ischium (*wark*);
- *Inferomedial*: the acetabular part (*ḥaqq al-fakhidh*), whose *deep cup* receives the *rounded head of the femur*.

Upon these bones are placed *noble organs*: the *bladder*, *uterus*, the *vessels of semen* in males, the *rectum* and *anus*.

Chapter Twenty-Six: General Function of the Leg (al-Rijl)

In sum, the leg serves *two ends*:

1. *Standing and support*—the *foot* is the chief organ of *stance*;
2. *Locomotion* on the *level, up, and down*—the *thigh* and *leg* are the principal movers.

If the *foot* is injured, *posture and steadiness* are impaired more than *locomotion* (beyond what transfer of weight to the other limb permits). If the *thigh and leg muscles* are injured, *standing is easy* but *movement is difficult*.

Chapter Twenty-Seven: The Femur (ʿAẓm al-Fakhidh)

The *femur* is the *largest bone* in the body: it *bears what is above* and *conveys what is below*. Its *proximal end* is *domed* to fit the *acetabular cup*. The shaft is *convex laterally* and *concave medially and posteriorly*:

- Were it laid *straight* in line with the cup, there would be a kind of *genu valgum* and poor *shelter* for the *great muscles*, *nerves*, and *vessels*, and the whole limb would lack *true straightness*, nor would the *sitting posture* be good.
- If it did not then *turn inward* again, a *different bow-leggedness* would appear and the *balance of stance* would not be right, nor the *inclination to and from the midline* well governed.

At its *distal end* are *two condyles* for the *knee joint*. We shall speak first of the *leg*, then of the *joint*.

Chapter Twenty-Eight: The Leg (al-Sāq)

Like the forearm, the *leg* has **two bones**:

- A *larger, longer, medial* bone—the **great shank** (*al-qaṣabah al-kubrā*; tibia)—the *true leg*;
- A *smaller, shorter, lateral* bone—the **lesser shank** (*al-qaṣabah al-ṣughrā*; fibula)—which does *not* meet the femur, falling *short proximally*, but *distally* reaches the level of the tibia.

The leg bows *laterally* in its upper course, then *medially* near the ankle—an arrangement that *betters balance and uprightness*. The *tibia* is *smaller than the femur*: the leg required both *greater size* (for *support and bearing*) and *greater smallness* (for *lightness and motion*). Since *lightness* is more crucial for the *leg's* purpose and *mass* for the *thigh's*, the tibia was made *slenderer*, the femur *larger*. The tibia was given a *measured thickness*:

- If *too great*, movement would be *encumbered* (as in *elephantiasis* or *varicose* swelling);
- If *too slight*, there would be *weakness*, impaired movement, and *inability to bear the upper weight* (as in naturally *stick-thin shanks*).

The *fibula buttresses* and *strengthens* the tibia, *screens* the *nerves and vessels* that run between them, and *shares* with the tibia in the *ankle joint*, reinforcing the *hinge of dorsiflexion and plantarflexion*.

Chapter Twenty-Nine: The Knee Joint (Mafṣal al-Rukbah)

The knee is formed by the entry of the two femoral condyles into their corresponding surfaces and is braced by a spiral encircling ligament, a deep binding ligament, and two strong collateral ligaments on either side. Its anterior aspect is completed by the patella—"the eye of the knee"—a nearly circular bone.

Functions of the patella: it shields the joint from tearing, dislocation, and wear during kneeling and the seat of support; it buttresses the joint as the body's weight is transferred over it in movement; and it is set in front because the most forceful bending occurs anteriorly (rising, kneeling, etc.). The knee does not bend violently backward, and its lateral motion is slight, while its principal flexion is forward, where the stresses lie.

Chapter Thirty: The Foot (al-Qadam)

The foot was fashioned as the organ of stance. Its shape is drawn forward to aid upright bearing, and it was given a medial arch (akhmaṣ) so that, especially in gait, the foot's tendency to erectness counters the outward tilt of the supporting limb, restoring balance. The arch also allows treading upon uneven, projecting ground without severe pain and lets the foot span steps and stair edges.

The foot is built from many bones. This yields secure grasp of the ground when needed—the foot can clasp a surface as the hand clasps an object—and a general advantage wherever bones are numerous, in that local injury does not disable the whole.

Count and plan (26 bones): talus (kaʿb), completing the joint with the leg; calcaneus (ʿaqib), the chief pillar of support; navicular (zawraqī), forming the arch; four tarsals that link to the metatarsus, one of which is the cuboid (nardī, die-like, hexagonal) on the lateral side, firming that side's purchase on the ground; and five metatarsals.

Talus. In humans it is more cubic than in other animals, the noblest foot bone for motion just as the calcaneus is the noblest for support. It lies between the malleoli of the two leg bones, which clasp it above, behind, and on both sides. Its ends are fixed into two sockets of the calcaneus. The talus is the intermediary between leg and heel: it secures their union and prevents wobble. Although the medial arch can make it seem shifted laterally, the talus is truly central. Anteriorly it articulates with the navicular.

Navicular. Posteriorly it meets the calcaneus; anteriorly, three tarsals (the cuneiforms); laterally, the cuboid (counted either as a separate bone or as the fourth of the distal tarsals).

Calcaneus. Set beneath the talus, hard and rounded posteriorly to resist blows; smooth inferiorly for a level plantar contact in standing. Its size is fitted to bear the body's weight. It is triangular and elongated, tapering toward the arch and slanting laterally so that the plantar concavity is formed gradually from heel toward midfoot.

Tarsus versus carpus. The tarsus has one row and fewer bones; the carpus has two rows and more parts. The hand needs mobility and enveloping; the foot, chiefly stability. Too many parts and joints weaken hold by excess looseness; too few remove the moderate yielding needed for proper placement. Hence many small parts suit grasping, while fewer, larger parts suit support.

Metatarsus and toes. Five metatarsals, one for each digit, arranged in a single row because the foot needs firmness more than the hand's cupping grasp. Each toe except the hallux has three phalanges; the hallux has two.

Grand total. Count all the bones and they are 248, excluding the sesamoids and the lambda-shaped bone corresponding to the Greek letter (the hyoid).

The Second Division: The Muscles (al-ʿaḍal)

Containing thirty chapters.

Chapter One: Nerves, Muscles, Tendons, and Ligaments

Since voluntary movement occurs only through a power that flows from the brain to the organs by way of the nerves, and since nerves by their delicate texture cannot attach directly to bones—which are in truth the first foundations of the organs that move by primary intention—the Creator, exalted be His wisdom, caused from the bones to sprout something resembling nerve substance. This is called the tendon (*ʿaqb*) or ligament (*ribāṭ*). It is joined with the nerve, interwoven with it as one structure.

Yet because the combined tissue of nerve and ligament remains fine and slender, for the nerve does not keep the full thickness it has at its origin, the All-wise Designer thickened it by mingling its fibers with flesh and enclosing the whole in a sheath, placing within it a central cord of nervous substance, like an axis. The resulting organ—composed of nerve, tendon, flesh, and covering membrane—is the muscle (*ʿaḍlah*).

When the muscle contracts, it draws the tendon attached to it along the side of the moving part, causing the limb to tighten and draw up. When it relaxes, the tendon slackens and the limb extends or moves away.

Chapter Two: Muscles of the Face

The muscles of the face correspond in number to its moving parts, which are: the forehead, the eyes, the upper eyelids, the cheeks (partly shared with the lips), and the lips themselves together with their two corners.

Chapter Three: Muscles of the Forehead

The forehead moves by means of a thin, broad, membranous muscle spread beneath the skin and intimately fused with it, almost forming part of the skin's own substance. It cannot be separated from it by scraping. This muscle meets its moving surface directly, without a tendon, for the part moved—the skin itself—is broad and light and not fit to be moved by a tendon. By its action, the eyebrows rise; by its relaxation, the eyelids assist the eye in closing.

Chapter Four: Muscles of the Eyeball (al-muqlah)

The eyeball is moved by six muscles: four placed on its four sides—above, below, at the inner and outer angles—each moving the eye in its own direction, and two oblique muscles that produce circular or rotational motion. Behind the eyeball lies another muscle supporting the hollow nerve sheath to which it is attached, preventing the eye from protruding and holding it steady during gaze. The membranes of this supporting muscle are so interwoven with ligamentous tissue that some anatomists regard it as a single muscle, while others divide it differently.

Chapter Five: Muscles of the Eyelid

The lower eyelid needs no muscle, for the purpose is fulfilled by motion of the upper lid alone. The divine wisdom always tends to minimize the number of instruments when the function can be achieved without loss. Though it is possible in theory for the lower lid to move and the upper to rest, the design follows a more direct order—bringing action close to its source. The upper lid is nearer the origin of the nerves; the nerve reaches it without winding or reversal.

Since the upper lid requires two movements—rising in opening and descending in closing—and since closing needs a muscle that pulls downward, a nerve approaches it obliquely from above. Were there only one such muscle, it would either attach to the middle or to one edge: if to the middle, it would draw the lid upward and obscure the pupil; if to one edge, the closure would be uneven. Therefore two equal muscles arise, one from each corner, drawing the lid downward symmetrically.

For lifting the lid, one muscle suffices. It descends straight between two membranes and spreads its tendon along the margin of the lid so that when it contracts, the lid opens. This tendon lies over a cartilaginous strip beneath the base of the eyelashes.

Chapter Six: Muscles of the Cheek

The cheek has two movements: one dependent on the lower jaw, the other shared with the lips. The first follows another organ's motion; the second it performs in partnership. The muscle responsible for this second motion is one broad sheet on each side of the face, each composed of four groups of fibers arising from four origins.

The first arises from the clavicle and ends at the corners of the mouth, pulling the lips downward. The second begins from the chest and the clavicle on both sides; its fibers cross obliquely so that those from the right attach to the left corner of the mouth and those from the left to the right, constricting and protruding the lips when they contract, as two drawstrings would. The third originates near the acromion of the shoulder and attaches above the preceding muscle, drawing the lips sideways equally. The fourth begins from the spinous processes of the neck, passes by the ears, and attaches to the cheek, moving it visibly together with the lips. In some persons its fibers come so near the ear's root that the ear itself moves when they act.

Chapter Seven: Muscles of the Lips

Some lip muscles are shared with the cheek; others belong to the lips alone. Four suffice: two descending from above along the lines of the cheeks to near the corners of the mouth, and two ascending from below. Each, acting singly, draws its half of the lip in its direction; acting in pairs, they spread the lips sideways, providing the four necessary movements. The tendons of these four, together with the ends of the shared muscles, are so blended with the substance of the lips that sensation cannot distinguish them from the lip's own flesh, since the lips are soft, fleshy parts without bone.

Chapter Eight: Muscles of the Nostrils

At the sides of the nasal tip are two small but strong muscles. Their smallness leaves room for the other facial muscles more constantly needed, for movements of the cheeks and lips are more frequent and essential. Yet they were made strong so that by force they compensate for the absence of bone. They arise from the region of the cheeks, interwoven at first with their fibers, and approach the nostrils from those sides because the motion they produce is toward them.

Chapter Nine: Muscles of the Lower Jaw

The lower jaw alone was given motion, for good reasons. First, it is better to move the lighter part. Second, it is safer to move what is less involved with delicate organs, since motion of the upper jaw would disturb many noble parts. Third, if the upper jaw were mobile, its joint with the head could not be firmly secured.

The jaw needs only three general movements: opening, closing, and side-to-side grinding. The opener lowers it; the closer raises it; the grinder moves it laterally.

Hence closure requires muscles descending from above that contract upward; opening needs muscles pulling downward; and grinding requires oblique ones. For closing, two muscles arise on each side, known as the temporal muscles (ʿaḍlat al-ṣudgh), lying beneath the temples. They are relatively small in humans because the moving part—the lower jaw—is light, and its motions gentle. In other animals, where the jaw is heavier, these muscles are larger and stronger, serving in biting and tearing.

These temporal muscles are soft near their origin in the brain, whose substance is tender. To protect them and prevent afflictions that might transmit to the brain, the Creator concealed their origins within the paired bones of the skull, channeling their fibers through arched passages until they emerge near the jaw, their substance gradually toughened by distance from the origin. Each produces a large tendon that grasps the edge of the jaw, so that contraction lifts it.

They are aided by two internal muscles descending within the mouth to the lower jaw, since the upward movement of a heavy part requires reinforcement. The tendon of each arises from the middle of the muscle for greater strength.

The muscles that open the mouth descend from the styloid processes behind the ears, join as one, then divide again, each becoming fleshy before attaching to the jaw near the chin. Their contraction draws the jaw backward and downward, lowering the mouth. Two suffice for this, aided by the natural downward tendency of the jaw.

For chewing there are also two muscles on each side, triangular in form, one angle at the cheekbone, from which extend two limbs: one descending to the jaw, the other ascending toward the temple, joined by a straight base between them. Each angle grips what lies near it, giving the muscle varied directions of contraction so its movement is not uniform but capable of different inclinations.

Chapter Ten: Muscles of the Head

The head performs its own specific movements and also shared movements together with five cervical vertebrae, producing coordinated motions of both head and neck. Each movement—whether specific or shared—may be forward bending, backward bending, or tilting to the right or to the left. From these combinations arises the rotary turning of the head.

The muscles that bend the head forward alone are two, arising on opposite sides. Their fibers attach above and behind the ears and below to the bones of the chest; they ascend as if conjoined—so much so that one might take them as a single muscle, or as two, or even as three when one branch divides into two heads. If one acts alone, the head bends forward and toward that side; if both act together, the head bends straight forward.

The muscles that bend head and neck forward together are a paired set lying beneath the esophagus, tapering toward the first and second vertebrae and attaching there. If the portion near the esophagus contracts, the head alone bends; if the portion fixed to the two vertebrae acts, the neck bends.

The muscles that throw the head backward alone are four pairs concealed beneath the foregoing. They arise above the joint: some from the spinous processes, with origins farther from the midline; others from the transverse processes, with origins closer to it. Thus: one pair comes to the wings of the first vertebra above; a second to the spine of the second vertebra; a third sends fibers from the wing of the first to the spine of the second, correcting lateral tilt when the head returns to the natural position; and a fourth begins above, passes under the third obliquely outward, and attaches to the wing of the first vertebra. The first two pairs extend the head backward without, or with only slight, tilt; the third rectifies inclination; the fourth extends with a clear obliquity. If either the third or fourth acts alone, the head inclines toward that side; if both act together, the head goes straight back without tilt.

The muscles that extend both head and neck are three deep pairs and one superficial pair. Each member of the superficial pair is triangular, its base fixed to the occipital bone and its apex descending onto the neck. Of the three deeper pairs beneath it: one descends along the sides of the vertebral column; one runs strongly toward the transverse processes; and one lies intermediate between the column's sides and the ends of the transverse processes.

The muscles that incline the head to the sides are two pairs that embrace the atlanto-occipital joints. One pair lies in front, joining the head to the second vertebra—one to the right, one to the left. The other pair lies behind, joining the head to the first vertebra—again one right, one left. Any one of these four, contracting alone, inclines the head toward its side with a slight obliquity. Any two on the same side incline the head to that side without obliquity. If the anterior pair acts, it assists forward bending; if the posterior pair acts, it assists backward bending. If all four act together, the head rises upright.

These four are the smallest of the muscles here, but their advantage lies in position and protection beneath larger muscles, compensating for what they lack in bulk. The head's joint needed two contrary provisions: firmness—secured by tight binding and little compliance—and multiplicity of movements—secured by laxity. Excellence of joint laxity was reconciled with firmness by the abundant twining of muscles around it. Thus both aims were achieved—blessed is God, best of creators and Lord of the worlds.

Chapter Eleven: Muscles of the Larynx

The larynx is a cartilaginous organ fashioned as the instrument of voice. It consists of three cartilages: first, the one palpable at the front of the throat beneath the chin, called the thyroid or shield, concave within and convex without like a buckler; second, a cartilage below it attached to the neck—"the unnamed" cartilage; third, a cartilage set over both, attached to the unnamed one and meeting the thyroid without direct union. Between this third cartilage and the unnamed one there is a double joint: two hollows receive two processes from the unnamed cartilage, bound by ligaments. This third cartilage is called the cricoid/epiglottic complex (here termed al-makkī or ṭarjahārī). By approaching or separating the thyroid and the unnamed cartilage, the laryngeal space narrows or widens. By folding the epiglottic piece over the thyroid and adhering to it—or withdrawing from it—the laryngeal inlet closes or opens.

In front of the larynx lies a triangular bone, the hyoid, named for its likeness to the Greek letter lambda. Its function is to provide a firm point of attachment from which laryngeal muscles arise.

The larynx needs: muscles that draw the thyroid toward the unnamed cartilage; muscles that draw and press down the epiglottis to close; and muscles that pull the epiglottis away to open. Among the openers are a pair arising from the hyoid, reaching and spreading upon the front of the thyroid; when they contract, they bring the epiglottic piece forward and upward and so enlarge the laryngeal space. Another pair—often counted among the tracheal muscles that draw downward—arises from the posterior chest and attaches to the thyroid; we include them among the shared muscles.

In many animals there is also another pair, and two further pairs: one reaching the epiglottis from behind—when they contract, they lift and pull it backward, disengaging it from the thyroid and widening the larynx; and one attaching to its edges—when they contract, they separate it from the thyroid laterally, helping to expand the opening.

Among the constrictors is a pair arising from near the hyoid, attaching to the thyroid, then passing transversely around the unnamed cartilage until their ends meet behind it; their contraction narrows the lumen. There are also four muscles (sometimes taken as two doubled muscles) spanning between the edges of the thyroid and the unnamed cartilage; when they act, they narrow the lower part of the larynx, some being internal and some external.

As for the closers, their best position is within the larynx so that on contracting they draw the epiglottic piece downward to shut the inlet. Thus there is a pair arising from the base of the thyroid, ascending internally to the margins of the epiglottis and to the base of the unnamed cartilage right and left. When they contract, they tighten the joint and firmly close the larynx, resisting the chest muscles and diaphragm in holding the breath. They are small so as not to narrow the lumen, yet strong to compensate for their size in the strenuous task of closure. Their course is mostly straight upward with slight obliquity to reach between the thyroid and the unnamed cartilage. Sometimes two additional muscles beneath the epiglottis assist this pair.

Chapter Twelve: Muscles of the Trachea and Pharynx

Taken together, the trachea has two pairs of muscles that draw it downward: one pair already mentioned with the larynx, and another pair also arising from the chest, ascending to the hyoid and then to the trachea, pulling it down. As for the pharynx, its muscles are the two palatal pillars (the "uvular arches"), set at the throat to assist swallowing. Know this.

Chapter Thirteen: Muscles of the Hyoid Bone

The hyoid has muscles peculiar to it and others shared. The exclusive set comprises three pairs: one from the sides of the mandible attaching to the straight ridge on the bone—this draws the hyoid toward the jaw; a second from beneath the chin passing under the tongue to the upper part of the bone—also drawing it toward the jaw; and a third from the styloid processes near the ears attaching to the lower end of the bone's straight ridge. Shared muscles have been mentioned and will be mentioned where appropriate.

Chapter Fourteen: Muscles of the Tongue

The tongue is moved by nine muscles: two transverse (from the styloid processes to the sides of the tongue); two longitudinal (from the upper hyoid to the root); two oblique (from the lesser horn of the hyoid, passing within the tongue between the longitudinal and the transverse sets); two flatteners/inverters beneath these, their fibers spreading broadly under the tongue and attaching across the mandible; and, counted with the tongue's ensemble, one unpaired muscle linking the tongue to the hyoid, drawing one to the other. It is not far-fetched that the muscle which lengthens the tongue toward prominence also moves it thus, for a muscle may act by extension as well as by shortening and contraction.

Chapter Fifteen: Muscles of the Neck

The muscles that move the neck alone are two pairs: one on the right, one on the left. If a single one acts, the neck is drawn toward that side obliquely; if both on the same side act together, the neck inclines straight to that side without obliquity; if all four act, the neck becomes upright without tilt.

Chapter Sixteen: Muscles of the Chest

The muscles that move the chest include those that expand it only and those that contract it only, as well as those that assist both motions.

Among the expanders is the diaphragm, the partition between the organs of respiration and the organs of digestion, which will be described later. Another pair lies beneath the clavicles, originating from a portion extending toward the head of the shoulder, half of it lying at some distance, and attached to the first rib on both sides. A third pair, each member double, has an upper part connecting with the neck—moving it—and a lower part that moves the chest. It is associated with another muscle attached to the fifth and sixth ribs. A further pair lies deep within the concave region of the shoulder, joined with a pair descending from the vertebrae to the shoulder, together forming one composite muscle attached to the posterior ribs. A third pair originates from the seventh cervical and the first and second thoracic vertebrae, attaching to the ribs near the sternum. These are the principal expanding muscles.

The contracting muscles of the chest include those that act transversely and those that act directly. The diaphragm, when it relaxes, contracts the thoracic cavity transversely. Another pair, stretched beneath the upper ribs, draws them together. Yet another pair, near the sternum between the xiphoid and clavicle, lies adjacent to the rectus abdominis, aided by two additional pairs.

Those muscles that act in both expansion and contraction are the intercostal muscles. Closer study shows that the flexors and extensors among them are distinct, for between every two ribs there are in fact four muscles, though they appear as one. What seems a single intercostal layer is woven of oblique fibers—some lying deep, some superficial. The superficial set includes two groups: one near the cartilaginous ends of the ribs and another near the bony ends. The deep set lies opposite to these in direction. Thus, the fiber patterns being four, the muscles themselves are four: those above serve to expand, and those below to contract. In total, the chest muscles number eighty-eight.

Two additional muscles aid the expansion of the chest. They arise from the clavicle and insert into the head of the shoulder, raising the first rib and thus contributing to chest elevation and expansion.

Chapter Seventeen: Muscles Moving the Arm (al-ʿaḍud)

The muscles that move the arm at the shoulder joint include several that draw it downward, upward, or backward.

Three muscles arise from the chest and pull the arm downward. One originates below the breast, attaching to the front of the humerus near the head beneath the clavicle; it draws the arm toward the chest while also depressing it, carrying the shoulder downward. A second arises from the upper sternum and passes inward to the head of the humerus, drawing it toward the chest with a slight lift. A third, large and double-headed, arises from the whole sternum and attaches below the front of the humerus; its upper fibers draw the arm toward the chest and upward, its lower fibers draw it downward, and together they move it straight toward the body.

Two other muscles arise from the flank. One, large and strong, originates near the loins and the posterior ribs, pulling the arm backward toward the ribs. The other, smaller and thinner, arises from the soft tissues of the flank rather than bone, inclining more toward the midline, and attaches deep to the tendon of the great pectoral muscle; it assists the first, drawing slightly backward.

Five muscles originate from the scapula.
—One arises between the scapular spine and its upper ridge, inserting into the upper outer part of the humeral head with a slight inward inclination; it lifts the arm outward and upward.
—Two arise from the upper ridge of the scapula: the first, large, sends fibers to the lower parts of the scapular spine and attaches to the outermost side of the humeral head, drawing it away from the body; the second, closely joined with the first as if part of it, attaches obliquely to the humerus, aiding in abduction.
—The fourth occupies the concave inner surface of the scapula, its tendon attaching to the medial side of the humeral head, turning the arm backward.
—The fifth arises from the lower end of the scapula's inferior border, its tendon attaching above the insertion of the large muscle ascending from the flank; it pulls the upper head of the arm upward.

The arm also has a two-headed muscle performing two distinct actions and a shared one. It arises from beneath the clavicle and from the neck, grasping the head of the humerus near the tendon of the pectoral muscle. One head lies internal, slanting inward;

the other external, from the back of the shoulder below, slanting outward. Acting together, they raise the arm straight upward. Some individuals possess two additional small muscles, one arising from the breast and another accompanying it.

Chapter Eighteen: Muscles Moving the Forearm (al-sāʿid)

The muscles that move the forearm include flexors, extensors, pronators (turning the palm down), and supinators (turning it up).

The extensors are a pair: one member extends the forearm with a slight inward inclination, arising from beneath the front of the arm and the lower scapular ridge, inserting on the inner side of the elbow; the other extends with a slight outward inclination, arising from the posterior humerus and inserting on the outer side of the elbow. Acting together, they extend the forearm straight.

The flexors are also a pair. The larger flexes with inward inclination, arising from the lower scapula and coracoid process, each origin forming a separate head; their tendon, fibrous in texture, attaches to the front of the upper ulna. The second flexor acts with outward inclination, arising from the posterior and outer surface of the humerus. It too is double-headed, one fleshy head behind and one before the bone, passing beneath it toward the front of the lower ulna. The inner flexor attaches higher, the outer lower, securing a firm and balanced pull. When both contract together, the forearm bends straight without deviation. Beneath the extensors lies another smaller muscle encircling the humerus, sometimes mistaken for part of the last flexor.

The pronators, which turn the forearm downward, form a pair. One lies externally between the two forearm bones, meeting the upper ulna without a tendon. The other, thin and elongated, arises from the upper external humerus and runs through the forearm nearly to the wrist, attaching by a membranous tendon to the inner side of the upper ulna.

The supinators, which turn the forearm upward, are also a pair. One arises from the upper inner part of the humeral head and attaches to the upper radius short of the wrist joint. The other, shorter and more tendinous, arises from the lower ulna and attaches to the upper radius near the wrist joint, its transverse fibers turning the forearm upward.

Chapter Nineteen: Muscles Moving the Wrist

Muscles for wrist motion include flexors, extensors, pronators (kap), and supinators (baṭḥ to the back of the hand).

Among the extensors are two closely joined muscles. The first arises from the mid–ulna; its tendon goes to the thumb and abducts it from the index. The second arises from the radius; its tendon inserts on the first carpal (by the thumb). Together they extend the wrist with slight pronation; the second alone supinates (backs) the hand, and the first alone separates thumb from index.

Another extensor lies on the radial (lateral) side of the forearm, originating from the lower humerus. Its split tendon reaches the bases of the metacarpals of middle and index; where its tendon rides over the radius at the wrist it extends the wrist with some pronation.

Flexors: a pair on the lateral side of the forearm. The lower begins at the inner humeral head and ends at the little-finger metacarpal; the upper begins higher and ends at the same place. A companion flexor arises from the lower humerus between the two and has two crossing sheaths that unite and insert between index and middle. Acting together, these flex.

These same flexors and extensors also pronate/supinate when opposing obliquely. The metacarpal-side muscle to the little finger alone can turn the palm over; aided by the thumb muscle (below) it completes full supination. The carpal-side muscle in front of the thumb alone produces slight pronation; with the little-finger–side muscle it pronates fully.

Chapter Twenty: Muscles Moving the Fingers

Finger movers lie in the hand and in the forearm. Concentrating them all in the hand would overburden it with flesh, so many originate in the forearm; their long tendons are strengthened by sheaths on all sides. The tendons are round and strong, flattening only at their insertions for a better grip.

All finger extensors are on the forearm, as are the primary flexors.
An extensor on the dorsal mid-forearm arises from the lower humeral ridge and sends four tendons to extend the four fingers.

Flexors to draw fingers downward are three, contiguous laterally. One arises from the middle outer humeral ridge (between its two processes) and sends two tendons to ring and little fingers. A doubled pair (two of the three) arise from the inner humeral epicondyle and ulnar border, sending two tendons to middle and index. The third arises from the upper radius and sends a tendon to the thumb. Near it runs another muscle (counted with the wrist group) from mid-ulna whose tendon abducts the thumb from the index.

Forearm flexors: three stacked centrally. The deepest and chief begins on the inner side of the humerus, joins the lower ulna, then its tendon broadens and splits into five: one to each finger pad. The four for the fingers flex the first and third joints (first via a sling-like band, third by direct insertion). The thumb slip flexes its second and third joints.
Above it, a smaller second flexor starts from the inner humeral head, touches the ulna, courses along the superior surface of the radius, then turns inward near the thumb and sends slips to the middle joints of the four fingers (a small offshoot reaches the

thumb from another point). A third is not for flexion: its tendon spreads across the palm to add sensibility, prevent hair growth there, and reinforce the palmar hollow.

Intrinsic hand muscles are eighteen in two layers: a deep (inner) layer and a superficial (outer) layer under the skin. Deep/inner layer: seven. Five elevate (dorsiflex) the fingers; the thumb muscle of them springs from the first carpal. A short broad sixth with oblique fibers anchors on the metacarpal at the level of the middle finger and by its tendon draws the thumb downward. A seventh at the little finger arises from its metacarpal and draws it downward. None of these seven flex; five elevate, two depress. Superficial/outer layer (under the palmar aponeurosis): eleven. Eight are arranged as four pairs for the first joints of the four fingers—each pair stacked (a lower that flexes with depression, and an upper that flexes with slight elevation; together they flex straight). Three belong to the thumb: one flexes the first joint and two the second. Thus, stabilizers other than for thumb and little finger have one each; thumb and little finger have two each. Flexors per finger are four; dorsiflexors per finger are one.

Chapter Twenty-One: Muscles Moving the Spine

Spinal muscles either extend the trunk backward or flex it forward; other motions derive from these. The true "back muscles" are the extensors: two longitudinal columns, each likely composed of twenty-three segmental portions (one per vertebra except the first). Moderate contraction erects the spine; strong contraction arches it backward. Acting unilaterally they incline the trunk to that side.

Flexors: two pairs. The upper pair belong to the head/neck group running beside the esophagus; their lower ends attach to the upper four or five thoracic vertebrae, their upper to head and neck. The lower pair (the "metnayn") begin at the tenth and eleventh thoracic and descend, producing forward flexion. The mid-spine follows the motions of the two ends, so these suffice for overall bending and bowing.

Chapter Twenty-Two: Muscles of the Abdomen

Eight abdominal muscles share functions: assisting expulsion of stool, urine, and the fetus; supporting the diaphragm during forced expiration; and warming stomach and intestines.

A straight pair runs from the xiphoid region down to the pubis, fleshy throughout.
Two transverse muscles cross these, lying above the abdominal fascia and below the two verticals; their fibers intersect the verticals at right angles.
Two oblique pairs (right and left), each itself two criss-crossing layers: from ensiform to pubis and from flank to costal arch. The lower ends of these approach the midline as broad tendons like membranes where they meet the straight pair; they lie superficial to the vertical pair and the transverses.

Chapter Twenty-Three: Muscles of the Testes/Ovaries

In men there are four cremasteric muscles to support and elevate the testes, one pair per testis. In women, a single pair suffices since their gonads are not pendulous like those of men.

Chapter Twenty-Four: Muscle of the Bladder Neck

A single circular muscle encircles the bladder's outlet. Its function is continence until voluntary release; when it relaxes, the abdominal muscles compress the bladder to void.

Chapter Twenty-Five: Muscles of the Penis

Two pairs move the penis. One pair runs along its sides; when they tense, they widen and straighten the urethral passage to ease semen flow. The other pair arises from the pubis and inserts obliquely at the root; moderate contraction elevates and straightens the organ, stronger contraction tilts it backward; unilateral action tilts toward that side.

Chapter Twenty-Six: Muscles of the Anus

Four muscles. One encircles and intermingles densely with anal tissue like the lip muscle—closing the anus and squeezing out remnants. A second lies deeper and above it (toward the head), likely bifid, its ends attaching truly to the penile root. A third pair lies obliquely above all, lifting the rectum; prolapse follows relaxation.

Chapter Twenty-Seven: Muscles Moving the Thigh

Greatest are the extensors, then flexors, for standing depends chiefly on extension; next abductors, then adductors, then rotators.

Extensors: foremost is the largest muscle in the body, cloaking the ilium and ischium, wrapping the thigh from within and behind to the knee. With multiple origins, its portions produce varied actions: fibers from low pubis extend with medial bias; slightly higher fibers extend chiefly upward; much higher fibers extend with more medial bias; fibers from the ischium extend straight.

Another covers the hip joint posteriorly, with three heads (from flank, ischium, coccyx—two fleshy, one aponeurotic) and two insertions on the posterior femoral head; unilateral pull extends with tilt, bilateral extends straight.

Another springs from the outer ilium, inserting on the greater trochanter's top, extending with medial tilt; a similar one attaches first to the lesser trochanter below, then descends to act likewise but more slightly; there may be several from the lower outer ilium.

Another arises low on the ischium, slanting backward, extending with slight posterior and clear medial inclination.

Flexors: one straight muscle descends from two origins—end of the lumbar mass and the ilium—to the lesser trochanter medially, flexing with slight medial bias. Another from the pubis to the lower lesser trochanter; a third oblique alongside it, like a part of the great muscle; a fourth from the upright iliac spine, also drawing the leg while flexing the thigh.

Adductors inward: some already noted; another long one from pubis to the knee. Abductors outward: two, one from the broad iliac bone. Rotators: two; one arises from the lateral pubic side, the other medially; they course obliquely to meet and fuse near the hollow beside the back of the greater trochanter. Either alone rotates the thigh toward its side with slight extension.

Chapter Twenty-Eight: Muscles Moving the Leg and Knee

Three large anterior thigh muscles extend the knee. One of these is "doubled," with two heads (from the greater trochanter and from the front of the femur) and two terminations: a fleshy portion into the patella and a membranous slip to the medial femoral edge. The other two arise from the iliac septum and from the lateral femoral ridge; they unite into a single transverse tendon that encircles and secures the patella, then continues to the top of the tibia to extend the knee.

Flexors of the leg include a long narrow muscle from ilium and pubis (near the medial extensor) slanting to the inner side of the knee and attaching at the popliteal pit; it draws the leg up and medially. Three more—lateral, central, and medial—also flex: the lateral and central bias the pull outward; the medial, which starts at the ischial base, runs behind the thigh to the tibia's medial popliteal region (noted as greenish in color) and biases inward. A small "buried" popliteal muscle assists the central flexor. Some describe a slip from the doubled extensor's septal head that can help "cinch" the hip socket via a band.

Chapter Twenty-Nine: Muscles Moving the Ankle (Foot)

Dorsiflexors (lifters) include a large muscle in front of the medial tibia, arising from the lateral side of its head and coursing toward the great toe base to lift the foot; a second from the fibular head runs to the area near the little-toe base to lift as well—together producing straight dorsiflexion.

Plantarflexors (depressors) are a paired mass beginning from the femoral heads, filling the posterior leg and forming the great calcaneal tendon (Achilles) to the calcaneus; their oblique, slightly lateral pull stabilizes the foot on the ground. They're aided by a bluish-tinged muscle from the fibular head that stays fleshy to insert on the back of the calcaneus just above the main tendon. Injury to these or their tendon cripples gait. Another muscle splits to two tendons: one plantarflexes the foot via an insertion before the hallux, the other extends the big toe, drawing it slightly inward. Yet another arises from the lateral femoral head, briefly joins the calf group, then separates in the deep posterior leg to send a broad tendon under the sole, fanning out like the hand's palmar sheet for similar support.

Chapter Thirty: Muscles Moving the Toes

Foreleg flexors: one from the fibular head sends a tendon that splits to flex the middle and ring toes; a smaller one from the posterior leg splits to the little and index toes, then each branch gives a slip that unites into a single tendon to the big toe to flex it. A third, already noted between the tibiae, divides: one slip plantarflexes the foot, the other goes to the first joint of the great toe.

Intrinsic foot muscles in the sole include ten that earlier anatomists missed; Galen identified them. Each toe has a medial and lateral muscle that flex together straight or, singly, flex with an inward or outward bias. Four additional small muscles lie at the tarsus, one per toe, and there are two special flexors for hallux and little toe. These muscles intermix so intimately that injury to one weakens neighboring functions while they can partially substitute for one another—hence it's hard to flex some toes independently.

On the dorsum, five small muscles bias the toes outward (lateralward). On the plantar side, five counterparts link each toe to its medial neighbor, biasing them inward. With the two special muscles for hallux and little toe, this set mirrors the seven named groups.

The Harmony of Motion and Rest: Life as Systemic Balance

In *The Vital Spirit and the Network of Life*, Ibn Sīnā completes his portrayal of the human being as an interconnected system of structure and function, where every organ participates in a precise economy of energy and form. The bones, joints, and muscles described in *The System of Nature and the Balance of Life* are here enlivened by the currents of the *rūḥ ḥayawānī*—the vital spirit that moves through the vessels and nerves as light moves through air.

To Ibn Sīnā, life is motion governed by equilibrium. The heart does not merely pump blood—it maintains the rhythm of balance between heat and moisture, expansion and contraction. The nerves do not simply transmit impulses—they mediate between intention and action, will and embodiment. The organs of perception translate the world's forms into inner knowledge, uniting the physical and the intelligible.

In this volume, the *Canon* reveals the subtle logic of interdependence that defines Avicenna's medical cosmology. The vital, natural, and animal faculties (*quwā ḥayawāniyya, ṭabīʿiyya, and nafsāniyya*) form a triadic system through which being sustains itself. Each faculty operates through *work* (*ʿamal*)—the transformation of energy (*quwwah*) over time (*zamān*). The result is a dynamic homeostasis that anticipates the principles of systems theory: the idea that health is not static but a continual process of regulation and renewal.

By grounding physiology in the language of balance, Ibn Sīnā bridges the physical sciences and moral philosophy. The same principles that preserve bodily equilibrium also sustain social and cosmic harmony. Just as an excess of one humor disturbs the body, so too does excess in desire or power disturb the community. The physician, like the statesman, must restore proportion and order.

This second volume therefore stands not only as a document of medieval medical genius but as a philosophy of living systems. It illuminates how energy, motion, and organization cooperate to sustain existence—and how disruption of these relationships gives rise to disease, decay, and imbalance.

Together, these works affirm the vision that has guided this collection: that the study of life, whether in nature, the body, or society, is the study of systems that do *work* with *energy* across *time*. In this, Ibn Sīnā remains a teacher not of medicine alone, but of the universal logic that binds all things living.

— *End of Volume Two* —

Commentary — Volume 2

In this second volume, Ibn Sīnā reveals with profound clarity his view of the living body as a *system of systems* — a dynamic network sustained by motion, equilibrium, and the flow of vital energy. This volume advances beyond anatomical description to uncover the logic that binds every organ to every other. What appears to be a study of parts — the heart, the arteries, the brain, the nerves — is, in truth, an inquiry into the invisible system that unites them: the continuous circulation of *rūḥ ḥayawānī*, the vital spirit, through the entire organism.

For Ibn Sīnā, the body is not a collection of discrete structures, but a living unity animated by systemic correspondence. The heart gives rise to motion and heat; the brain refines and regulates perception; the liver sustains nourishment and growth. Each organ performs its own work (*ʿamal*), yet none can exist or act in isolation. Every pulse, every breath, every sensory act participates in a greater order of flow — a pattern of interdependence that mirrors the order of the cosmos itself.

The *rūḥ ḥayawānī* lies at the heart of this system. It is neither purely material nor purely immaterial, but an intermediary substance — a vehicle of energy bridging the physical and the spiritual. It circulates through arteries and nerves, carrying motion, perception, and life. In its function and form, it prefigures the modern concept of systemic regulation: a medium through which communication occurs among all parts of the organism. Ibn Sīnā's medical reasoning thus approaches what we would now call a *theory of complex systems* — a vision in which feedback, equilibrium, and adaptation define the conditions of health.

Throughout this volume, he weaves anatomy with philosophy, grounding the structure of the body in the metaphysical principles of balance and purpose. The organs are not mere instruments of life; they are expressions of universal design. Their harmony reflects the harmony of nature itself. The same proportional relationships that sustain the cosmos — between motion and rest, heat and cold, matter and form — also sustain the human being. The body is a microcosm whose inner order mirrors the outer order of creation.

Ibn Sīnā's insight lies in perceiving that *life is a process of mediation*: between heart and brain, between matter and spirit, between the human and the cosmic. He sees no divide between physiology and philosophy, between medicine and metaphysics. The systems of the body are extensions of the same natural logic that governs the heavens. The heart beats in rhythm with the stars; the breath echoes the movement of the air; the vital spirit circulates as the blood of the world itself.

Health is not simply the absence of disease — it is the perfect circulation of energy within the system and between systems. Disease arises when that circulation falters, when flow is obstructed or imbalanced. Healing, therefore, is the restoration of systemic harmony, not only within the organs but between the individual and the environment that sustains them.

This volume marks the turning point in Ibn Sīnā's *Canon*: the transition from the anatomy of the body to the philosophy of living systems. It prepares the way for *Volume 3*, where the focus shifts from the body's internal structures to the forces that act upon them — the rhythms of air, water, motion, and environment — showing that no system, however complete in itself, stands apart from the greater systems of nature.

Thus, Ibn Sīnā stands among the earliest thinkers to envision the human being as an *integrated system within a universal network of balance*. His medicine is not a science of isolation, but of connection — the art of perceiving how the pulse of the individual life participates in the rhythm of the world.

Glossary of Key Arabic Terms

Foundational / Philosophical Concepts

- rūḥ (روح) — vital spirit; animating principle of life
- rūḥ ḥayawānī — animal/vital spirit governing motion and sensation
- mizāj (مزاج) — temperament; balance of qualities (hot, cold, moist, dry)
- ṭabīʿa (طبيعة) — nature; intrinsic governing force of a body
- quwwa (قوة) — faculty, power, or capacity
- ʿamal (عمل) — action, function, or work performed by an organ
- zamān (زمان) — time (as a condition for processes)
- imtizāj (امتزاج) — mixture; blending of elements or humors
- gharīziyya (غريزية) — innate, natural, intrinsic

Structural Classification of Organs

- aʿḍāʾ (أعضاء) — organs
- aʿḍāʾ raʾīsiyya (أعضاء رئيسية) — principal organs
- aʿḍāʾ āliyya (أعضاء آلية) — instrumental organs
- mutashābih al-ajzāʾ (متشابه الأجزاء) — homogeneous organs
- khādimah (خادمة) — servant organs
- manfaʿa (منفعة) — benefit (preparatory function)
- khidma (خدمة) — service (executive function)
- fiʿl (فعل) — act or function

Core Anatomical Terms (General)

- ʿaẓm (عظم) — bone
- ʿiẓām (عظام) — bones

- ghuḍrūf (غضروف) — cartilage
- ʿaṣab (عصب) — nerve
- awtār (أوتار) — tendons
- rubāṭāt (رباطات) — ligaments
- ribāṭ (رباط) — binding ligament
- ʿaqb (عقب) — thick ligament (e.g., heel tendon)
- shiryānāt (شريانات) — arteries
- awrida (أوردة) — veins
- aghashiya (أغشية) — membranes
- laḥm (لحم) — flesh
- shaḥm (شحم) — fat

Physiological Processes

- quwwat al-ghidhāʾ (implicit) — nutritive faculty
- attraction / retention / expulsion / assimilation — described as faculties of nourishment
- al-ḥarāra al-gharīziyya — innate heat
- al-akhlāṭ (الأخلاط) — humors

Major Organs

- al-qalb (القلب) — heart
- al-dimāgh (الدماغ) — brain
- al-kabid (الكبد) — liver
- al-unthiyān (الأنثيان) — testicles
- al-riʾah (الرئة) — lung
- al-miʿda (المعدة) — stomach

Skeletal System (Selected Terms)

Spine and Axial Skeleton

- al-ṣulb (الصلب) — spine
- al-nukhāʿ (النخاع) — spinal cord
- al-kharza (الخرزة) — vertebra

- al-qaṭn (القطن) — lumbar region
- al-ʿajz (العجز) — sacrum
- al-ʿuṣʿuṣ (العصعص) — coccyx

Thoracic Structures

- al-aḍlāʿ (الأضلاع) — ribs
- al-qaṣ (القص) — sternum

Skull and Head Anatomy

- al-qaḥf (القحف) — skull
- ḥujratān (حجرتان) — temporal bones ("chambers")
- al-ʿaẓm al-watadī (العظم الوتدي) — sphenoid bone
- al-ṣifāq (الصفاق) — peritoneum

Upper Limb

- al-ʿaḍud (العضد) — upper arm
- ʿaẓm al-ʿaḍud — humerus
- al-sāʿid (الساعد) — forearm
- al-mirfaq (المرفق) — elbow
- al-rusrugh (الرسغ) — wrist
- mashṭ al-kaff (مشط الكف) — metacarpus
- al-aṣābiʿ (الأصابع) — digits
- al-ẓufr (الظفر) — nail

Lower Limb

- al-rijl (الرجل) — leg
- ʿaẓm al-fakhidh (عظم الفخذ) — femur
- al-sāq (الساق) — lower leg
- mafṣal al-rukbah (مفصل الركبة) — knee joint
- al-qadam (القدم) — foot

Joints and Structural Terms

- mafṣil (مفصل) — joint

- darz (درز) — suture (cranial joint)
- nuqar / nukr (نقر) — sockets or pits
- laqam (لقم) — condyloid projections

Sensory and Functional Anatomy

- al-muqlah (المقلة) — eyeball
- qaṣabat al-ri'ah (قصبة الرئة) — trachea

Reproductive and Developmental Terms

- al-maniy (مني) — semen
- al-dam al-ḥayḍ (حيض) — menstrual blood
- al-arbiyatān (الأربيتان) — groins
- Conceptual/Systemic Language
- niẓām (implicit) — system/order
- tawāzun (implicit) — balance
- ḥarakah (حركة) — motion
- sukūn (سكون) — rest

General Notes

The glossary confirms Ibn Sīnā's systemic vocabulary revolves around:

- quwwa (power)
- ʿamal (function/work)
- mizāj (balance/temperament)

There is a clear triadic structure:

- structure (ʿuḍw / organ)
- power (quwwa)
- action (fiʿl / ʿamal)

The terminology strongly supports the *systems-thinking framework*: organs are not isolated objects but nodes of action and exchange.

End of

The Architecture of the Body and the Order of Life

The Architecture of the Body and the Order of Life presents Ibn Sīnā's vision of the human body as an integrated system in which structure and function are inseparably joined. Beginning with the nature and classification of organs, he traces the hierarchy through which bones, tissues, and vital systems are arranged to sustain both life and motion. Each part is defined not merely by its form, but by its role—its *quwwa* (power) and *ʿamal* (action)—within a larger, ordered whole. In this account, anatomy becomes more than description; it is the study of a living architecture governed by balance (*mizāj*), coordination, and purpose, where the stability of the body and the continuity of life depend on the harmony of its parts. The selection is drawn from *Ibn Sīnā's Canon of Medicine* (*al-Qānūn fī al-Ṭibb*).

Ibn Sīnā (Avicenna, 980–1037 CE) conceived medicine as the applied art of maintaining equilibrium within the living body. To him, the physician was both a scientist and a philosopher of nature, charged not only with healing disease but with understanding the laws that govern vitality itself.

This translation presents that vision anew—faithful to his terminology, rigorous in structure, and accessible to readers of medicine, philosophy, and the sciences alike.

We invite you to immerse yourself in this selection and discover the depth and coherence of Ibn Sīnā's vision of the living body. Stay engaged as the editors of the Ancient Wisdom Collection continue to bring forward future volumes, each uncovering new dimensions of this enduring intellectual tradition.

www.ingramcontent.com/pod-product-compliance
Lightning Source LLC
LaVergne TN
LVHW051044210926
848486LV00001B/10
* 9 7 9 8 8 8 8 2 3 0 1 9 0 *